Prostate Cancer: Recent Advances in Diagnostics and Treatment Planning

Prostate Cancer: Recent Advances in Diagnostics and Treatment Planning

Guest Editor

Theodoros Tokas

MDPI

Basel • Beijing • Wuhan • Barcelona • Belgrade • Novi Sad • Cluj • Manchester

Guest Editor
Theodoros Tokas
Department of Urology
University General Hospital
of Heraklion
University of Crete
Medical School
Heraklion
Greece

Editorial Office
MDPI AG
Grosspeteranlage 5
4052 Basel, Switzerland

This is a reprint of the Special Issue, published open access by the journal *Journal of Clinical Medicine* (ISSN 2077-0383), freely accessible at: https://www.mdpi.com/journal/jcm/special_issues/Prostate_Cancer_JCM.

For citation purposes, cite each article independently as indicated on the article page online and as indicated below:

Lastname, A.A.; Lastname, B.B. Article Title. *Journal Name* **Year**, *Volume Number*, Page Range.

ISBN 978-3-7258-4295-7 (Hbk)
ISBN 978-3-7258-4296-4 (PDF)
https://doi.org/10.3390/books978-3-7258-4296-4

Contents

Journal of
Clinical Medicine

MDPI

Editorial

Special Issue "Prostate Cancer: Recent Advances in Diagnostics and Treatment Planning"

Theodoros Tokas [1,2]

[1] Department of Urology and Andrology, General Hospital Hall i.T., Milser Str. 10, 6060 Hall in Tirol, Austria; ttokas@yahoo.com; Tel.: +43-(0)50504-36310

[2] Training and Research in Urological Surgery and Technology (T.R.U.S.T.)-Group, Milser Str. 10, 6060 Hall in Tirol, Austria

This editorial of the Special Issue "Prostate Cancer: Recent Advances in Diagnostics and Treatment Planning" aims to draw more attention to the broad and diverse field of prostate cancer (PCa) diagnosis and the utilization of different diagnostic means to improve clinical decision-making and treatment strategy planning. PCa is the second most frequent malignancy in men [1]. Tumor aggressiveness varies, ranging from non-aggressive tumors that may be safely monitored to poor prognosis tumors only suited for palliative treatment. Undoubtedly, new imaging modalities such as magnetic resonance imaging (MRI) and positron emission tomography (PET) with targeted tracers are more sensitive than conventional imaging [2] and may result in stage migration and a natural inclination toward altering clinical management. In contrast to other cancers, the PCa community acknowledges that precision medicine has developed more slowly [3]. Genetic counseling and germline testing can aid in the early detection and management of PCa. Biomarkers based on urine, serum, and tissue increase PCa patient detection and facilitate risk stratification.

Indications for prostate biopsy can be determined with the aid of MRI, which is also essential for local staging. When combined with clinicopathological information, MRI results in a more accurate prognosis, which may help with tailored patient care [4]. In the case of localized PCa, MRI findings are associated with clinically relevant long-term oncologic outcomes. The diagnosis of clinically significant PCa is improved by targeted biopsies, as routine transrectal ultrasonography is not always accurate. Additionally, the evidence supporting the addition of MRI-targeted biopsies to systematic biopsies necessitates a review of the active surveillance (AS) inclusion criteria and a shift in research focus away from one-size-fits-all protocols and toward more flexible and personalized risk-based AS approaches [5]. On the other hand, modern, less expensive ultrasound-based techniques can deliver high-quality imaging in the absence of an MRI [6–8].

Prostate-specific membrane antigen (PSMA) PET has been adopted for staging aggressive tumors. Compared with traditional imaging, PSMA PET offers a reasonably good sensitivity for detecting regional and extrapelvic metastases. Additionally, it can play a significant part in the early diagnosis of extraprostatic disease and help with surgical planning. Furthermore, PSMA PET has been shown to be a valuable technique for planning definitive radiation therapy in patients who have not yet received treatment [9]. Furthermore, even at low PSA levels, PSMA PET is highly effective at detecting and localizing post-treatment biochemical recurrence [10]. Molecular PET, in the post-radical prostatectomy setting, leads to management modifications to prepare patients for salvage radiotherapy by detecting lesions in anatomical locations not typically included in the usual postoperative radiotherapy fields [11]. Finally, PSMA-PET provides more accurate staging for nonmetastatic castrate-resistant PCa, among other applications. In particular, target expression evaluation for PSMA radioligand therapy and target localization for metastasis-directed therapy show potential. Future trials must clarify the potential for this diagnostic tool to translate it into an oncologic benefit [12].

Genetic alterations are associated with differential prognosis and clinical phenotypes in metastatic PCa. Blood biomarkers could assist clinicians in managing patients with localized disease and provide the most robust degree of evidence for predicting more aggressive Pca [13]. Liquid biopsies are valuable as a source of prognostic, predictive, and response biomarkers in PCa. Most clinical applications have been developed in the advanced metastatic setting. These minimally invasive tests can guide diagnosis and treatment selection [14]. However, before therapeutic adoption, newly discovered data on these putative predictive biomarkers must be confirmed in biomarker-driven randomized controlled trials [15].

Together, these methods produce risk calculators/nomograms that can predict the risk of developing cancer, the likelihood that the disease will be aggressive, and the likelihood that the patient will respond well to therapy [16,17]. However, we need to learn how to appropriately interpret them and to treat patients while keeping in mind the clinical objectives, such as overall survival, disease recurrence, and quality of life, that the treatment intended to attain. This can only be achieved with sufficiently large studies of patients who are followed up for a long time, even if they are observational studies. This can reduce side effects, expenses, and resource usage while minimizing the danger of over- or under-treating patients.

Funding: This research received no external funding.

Conflicts of Interest: The author declares no conflict of interest.

References

1. Mottet, N.; van den Bergh, R.C.; Briers, E.; Van den Broeck, T.; Cumberbatch, M.G.; De Santis, M.; Fanti, S.; Fossati, N.; Gandaglia, G.; Gillessen, S.; et al. EAU-EANM-ESTRO-ESUR-SIOG Guidelines on Prostate Cancer-2020 Update. Part 1: Screening, Diagnosis, and Local Treatment with Curative Intent. *Eur. Urol.* **2021**, *79*, 243–262. [CrossRef] [PubMed]
2. Hofman, M.S.; Lawrentschuk, N.; Francis, R.J.; Tang, C.; Vela, I.; Thomas, P.; Rutherford, N.; Martin, J.M.; Frydenberg, M.; Shakher, R.; et al. Prostate-specific membrane antigen PET-CT in patients with high-risk prostate cancer before curative-intent surgery or radiotherapy (proPSMA): A prospective, randomised, multicentre study. *Lancet* **2020**, *395*, 1208–1216. [CrossRef]
3. De Santis, M.; Mottet, N.; Cornford, P.; Gillessen, S. Precision Oncology for Metastatic Prostate Cancer: Translation into Practice. *Eur. Urol.* **2020**, *78*, 771–774. [CrossRef] [PubMed]
4. Wibmer, A.G.; Chaim, J.; Lakhman, Y.; Lefkowitz, R.A.; Nincevic, J.; Nikolovski, I.; Sala, E.; Gonen, M.; Carlsson, S.V.; Fine, S.W.; et al. Oncologic Outcomes after Localized Prostate Cancer Treatment: Associations with Pretreatment Prostate Magnetic Resonance Imaging Findings. *J. Urol.* **2021**, *205*, 1055–1062. [CrossRef] [PubMed]
5. Venderbos, L.D.; Luiting, H.; Hogenhout, R.; Roobol, M.J. Interaction of MRI and active surveillance in prostate cancer: Time to re-evaluate the active surveillance inclusion criteria. *Urol. Oncol.* **2021**. [CrossRef] [PubMed]
6. Lorusso, V.; Kabre, B.; Pignot, G.; Branger, N.; Pacchetti, A.; Thomassin-Piana, J.; Brunelle, S.; Gregori, A.; Salem, N.; Musi, G.; et al. Comparison Between Micro-Ultrasound and Multiparametric MRI Regarding the Correct Identification of Prostate Cancer Lesions. *Clin. Genitourin. Cancer* **2022**, *20*, e339–e345. [CrossRef] [PubMed]
7. Correas, J.M.; Halpern, E.J.; Barr, R.G.; Ghai, S.; Walz, J.; Bodard, S.; Dariane, C.; de la Rosette, J. Advanced ultrasound in the diagnosis of prostate cancer. *World J. Urol.* **2021**, *39*, 661–676. [CrossRef] [PubMed]
8. Lorusso, V.; Kabre, B.; Pignot, G.; Branger, N.; Pacchetti, A.; Thomassin-Piana, J.; Brunelle, S.; Nicolai, N.; Musi, G.; Salem, N.; et al. External validation of the computerized analysis of TRUS of the prostate with the ANNA/C-TRUS system: A potential role of artificial intelligence for improving prostate cancer detection. *World J. Urol.* 2022; *Online ahead of print*. [CrossRef] [PubMed]
9. Murthy, V.; Sonni, I.; Jariwala, N.; Juarez, R.; Reiter, R.E.; Raman, S.S.; Hope, T.A. The Role of PSMA PET/CT and PET/MRI in the Initial Staging of Prostate Cancer. *Eur. Urol. Focus* **2021**, *7*, 258–266. [CrossRef] [PubMed]
10. Keegan, N.M.; Bodei, L.; Morris, M.J. Seek and Find: Current Prospective Evidence for Prostate-specific Membrane Antigen Imaging to Detect Recurrent Prostate Cancer. *Eur. Urol. Focus* **2021**, *7*, 267–278. [CrossRef] [PubMed]
11. Valle, L.; Shabsovich, D.; de Meerleer, G.; Maurer, T.; Murphy, D.G.; Nickols, N.G.; Vapiwala, N.; Calais, J.; Kishan, A.U. Use and Impact of Positron Emission Tomography/Computed Tomography Prior to Salvage Radiation Therapy in Men with Biochemical Recurrence After Radical Prostatectomy: A Scoping Review. *Eur. Urol. Oncol.* **2021**, *4*, 339–355. [CrossRef] [PubMed]
12. Weber, M.; Hadaschik, B.; Ferdinandus, J.; Rahbar, K.; Bögemann, M.; Herrmann, K.; Fendler, W.P.; Kesch, C. Prostate-specific Membrane Antigen-based Imaging of Castration-resistant Prostate Cancer. *Eur. Urol. Focus* **2021**, *7*, 279–287. [CrossRef] [PubMed]

13. Lamy, P.J.; Allory, Y.; Gauchez, A.S.; Asselain, B.; Beuzeboc, P.; de Cremoux, P.; Fontugne, J.; Georges, A.; Hennequin, C.; Lehmann-Che, J.; et al. Prognostic Biomarkers Used for Localised Prostate Cancer Management: A Systematic Review. *Eur. Urol. Focus* **2018**, *4*, 790–803. [CrossRef] [PubMed]
14. Casanova-Salas, I.; Athie, A.; Boutros, P.C.; Del Re, M.; Miyamoto, D.T.; Pienta, K.J.; Posadas, E.M.; Sowalsky, A.G.; Stenzl, A.; Wyatt, A.W.; et al. Quantitative and Qualitative Analysis of Blood-based Liquid Biopsies to Inform Clinical Decision-making in Prostate Cancer. *Eur. Urol.* **2021**, *79*, 762–771. [CrossRef] [PubMed]
15. Van der Eecken, K.; Vanwelkenhuyzen, J.; Deek, M.P.; Tran, P.T.; Warner, E.; Wyatt, A.W.; Kwan, E.M.; Verbeke, S.; Van Dorpe, J.; Fonteyne, V.; et al. Tissue- and Blood-derived Genomic Biomarkers for Metastatic Hormone-sensitive Prostate Cancer: A Systematic Review. *Eur. Urol. Oncol.* **2021**, *4*, 914–923. [CrossRef] [PubMed]
16. Luzzago, S.; de Cobelli, O.; Cozzi, G.; Peveri, G.; Bagnardi, V.; Catellani, M.; Di Trapani, E.; Mistretta, F.A.; Pricolo, P.; Conti, A.; et al. A novel nomogram to identify candidates for active surveillance amongst patients with International Society of Urological Pathology (ISUP) Grade Group (GG) 1 or ISUP GG2 prostate cancer, according to multiparametric magnetic resonance imaging findings. *BJU Int.* **2020**, *126*, 104–113. [CrossRef] [PubMed]
17. Ma, M.W.; Gao, X.S.; Lyu, F.; Gu, X.B.; Yin, H.; Li, H.Z.; Li, X.Y.; Qi, X.; Bai, Y.; Chen, J.Y. Development of a nomogram predicting metastatic disease and the assessment of NCCN, AUA and EAU guideline recommendations for bone imaging in prostate cancer patients. *World J. Urol.* **2021**, *39*, 1815–1823. [CrossRef] [PubMed]

Journal of
Clinical Medicine

MDPI

Article

Could 68Ga-PSMA PET/CT Evaluation Reduce the Number of Scheduled Prostate Biopsies in Men Enrolled in Active Surveillance Protocols?

Pietro Pepe [1,*], Marco Roscigno [2], Ludovica Pepe [1], Paolo Panella [1], Marinella Tamburo [3], Giulia Marletta [3], Francesco Savoca [1], Giuseppe Candiano [1], Sebastiano Cosentino [4], Massimo Ippolito [4], Andreas Tsirgiotis [1] and Michele Pennisi [1]

[1] Urology Unit, Cannizzaro Hospital, 95126 Catania, Italy; ludopepe97@gmail.com (L.P.); ppanella5@gmail.com (P.P.); francescosavoca@virgilio.it (F.S.); urocandia@gmail.com (G.C.); tsirgiotis.andreas@gmail.com (A.T.); michepennisi2@virgilio.it (M.P.)

[2] Department of Surgery, UOC Urologia, ASST Papa Giovanni XXIII, 24127 Bergamo, Italy; roscigno.marco@gmail.com

[3] Radiotherapy Unit, Cannizzaro Hospital, 95126 Catania, Italy; marinella.tamburo@virgilio.it (M.T.); marlettagiulia1@gmail.com (G.M.)

[4] Nuclear Medicine Unit, Cannizzaro Hospital, 95126 Catania, Italy; ianocose@hotmail.com (S.C.); massimo.ippolito@aoec.it (M.I.)

* Correspondence: piepepe@hotmail.com; Tel.: +39-9-5726-3285; Fax: +39-9-5726-3259

Abstract: Background: To evaluate the accuracy of 68Ga-prostate specific membrane antigen (PSMA) PET/CT in the diagnosis of clinically significant prostate cancer (csPCa) (Grade Group > 2) in men enrolled in Active Surveillance (AS) protocol. Methods: From May 2013 to May 2021, 173 men with very low-risk PCa were enrolled in an AS protocol study. During the follow-up, 38/173 (22%) men were upgraded and 8/173 (4.6%) decided to leave the AS protocol. After four years from confirmatory biopsy (range: 48–52 months), 30/127 (23.6%) consecutive patients were submitted to mpMRI and 68Ga-PSMA PET/CT scan before scheduled repeated biopsy. All the mpMRI (PI-RADS > 3) and 68Ga-PET/TC standardised uptake value (SUVmax) > 5 g/mL index lesions underwent targeted cores (mpMRI-TPBx and PSMA-TPBx) combined with transperineal saturation prostate biopsy (SPBx: median 20 cores). Results: mpMRI and 68Ga-PSMA PET/CT showed 14/30 (46.6%) and 6/30 (20%) lesions suspicious for PCa. In 2/30 (6.6%) men, a csPCa was found; 68Ga-PSMA-TPBx vs. mpMRI-TPBx vs. SPBx diagnosed 1/2 (50%) vs. 1/2 (50%) vs. 2/2 (100%) csPCa, respectively. In detail, mpMRI and 68Ga-PSMA PET/TC demonstrated 13/30 (43.3%) vs. 5/30 (16.7%) false positive and 1 (50%) vs. 1 (50%) false negative results. Conclusion: 68Ga-PSMA PET/CT did not improve the detection for csPCa of SPBx but would have spared 24/30 (80%) scheduled biopsies showing a lower false positive rate in comparison with mpMRI (20% vs. 43.3%) and a negative predictive value of 85.7% vs. 57.1%, respectively.

Keywords: prostate cancer; 68Ga-PSMA PET/CT; mpMRI; targeted prostate biopsy; active surveillance

1. Introduction

In the last decade, active surveillance (AS) has become an alternative to radical treatment of low-/very low-risk prostate cancer (PCa), focusing on prevention of overtreatment (50% of the cases in screening studies) [1–3]. Multiparametric magnetic resonance imaging (mpMRI) has demonstrated good accuracy in diagnosing clinically significant PCa (csPCa), particularly if the cancer is located in the anterior prostate [4]; therefore, mpMRI is now strongly recommended in AS follow-up [5]. However, the time of confirmatory biopsy has been established within one year from initial diagnosis [6], and there are no data regarding the number of systematic needle cores and the best imaging procedure to use for omitting or postponing scheduled repeated biopsies.

Recently, prostate-specific membrane antigen (PSMA) inhibitors conjugated with the radionuclides 68Ga and 18F-fluoride have been well-explored and successfully translated for the clinical diagnosis of PCa [7,8]. Moreover, tumour uptake, which represents PSMA expression, results were highly correlated with the Gleason score of the primary prostatic tumour [9]. However, in a limited number of studies focused on the primary prostatic lesion, 68Ga-PSMA positron emission tomography/computed tomography (PET/CT) has been shown to be sensitive for the detection of primary prostatic lesions and regional lymphadenopathy [10–12]. Recently, Raveethiran et al. suggested that the addition of a diagnostic 68Ga-PSMA PET/CT to mpMRI can improve the detection of significant prostate cancer and improve the ability to identify men suitable for active surveillance [13].

The aim of this study was to prospectively evaluate the diagnostic accuracy of 68Ga-PSMA PET/CT and mpMRI in the diagnosis of csPCa (Grade Group > 2) [14] in men enrolled in AS protocol.

2. Materials and Methods

From May 2013 to May 2021, 173 men aged between 52 and 73 (median age 63) with very low-risk PCa were enrolled in an AS protocol study. After institutional review board and ethical committee approval were granted, informed consents were obtained from all participants included in the study. Presence of the following criteria defined eligibility: life expectancy greater than 10 years, clinical stage T1C, PSA below 10 ng/mL, PSA density (PSA-D) < 0.20, <2 unilateral positive biopsy cores, Gleason score 6/International Society of Urologic Pathology (ISUP) Grade Groups (GG) 1 [14] and maximum core percentage of cancer (GPC) < 50% (3). All the patients underwent confirmatory biopsy six months after the PCa diagnosis and mpMRI evaluation. During the follow-up, 38/173 (22%) men were upgraded and 8/173 (4.6%) men autonomously decided to leave the AS protocol. After four years from confirmatory biopsy (range: 48–52 months), also in the presence of stable clinical parameters, the last 30/127 (23.6%) consecutive patients were submitted to mpMRI and 68Ga-PET/CT imaging examinations before scheduled repeated biopsy.

All mpMRI examinations were performed using a 3.0 Tesla scanner (ACHIEVA 3T; Philips Healthcare, Best, The Netherlands) equipped with 16 surface channel phased-array coils placed around the pelvic area with the patient in the supine position; multi-planar turbo spin-echo T2-weighted (T2W), axial diffusion weighted imaging (DWI) and axial dynamic contrast enhanced (DCE) were performed for each patient. The mpMRI lesions characterised by Prostate Imaging Reporting and Data System (PI-RADS) version 2 (4) scores > 3 were considered suspicious for cancer; two radiologists blinded to pre-imaging clinical parameters evaluated the mpMRI data separately and independently; moreover, one urologist with more than 25 years of experience performed the biopsy procedure [6]. The data were collected following the Screening Tool to Alert to Right Treatment (START) criteria [15].

PET/CT imaging was performed using a CT-integrated PET scanner (Biograph 6; Siemens, Knoxville, TN, USA). 68Ga-PSMA was prepared with a fully automated radiopharmaceutical synthesis device based on a modular concept (Eckert & Ziegler Eurotope, Berlin, Germany). 68Ga-PSMA-11 was given to patients via an intravenous bolus (mean, 144 $\pm$ 12 MBq; range, 122–188 MBq), and the PET acquisition was started at a mean of 58 $\pm$ 12 min (range, 50–81 min) afterward. Scans were acquired in 3-dimensional mode with an acquisition time of 3 min per bed position. Emission data were corrected for randoms, dead time, scatter and attenuation and were reconstructed iteratively using ordered-subsets expectation maximisation (4 iterations, 8 subsets) followed by a post-reconstruction smoothing Gaussian filter (5 mm in full width at half maximum). For attenuation correction, a low-dose unenhanced CT scan was performed from the skull base to the middle of the thigh. Images were processed to obtain PET, CT, and PET-CT fusion sections in the axial, coronal, and sagittal planes with a thickness of approximately 0.5 cm by two experienced nuclear medicine specialists, who were blinded to the clinical data. The location of focal uptake on 68Ga-PSMA PET/CT (Figure 1), three-dimensional size, and standardised uptake value (SUVmax) values were reported on a per-lesion basis with a sexstant scheme (apex, midgland and base, each split into left and right) [7].

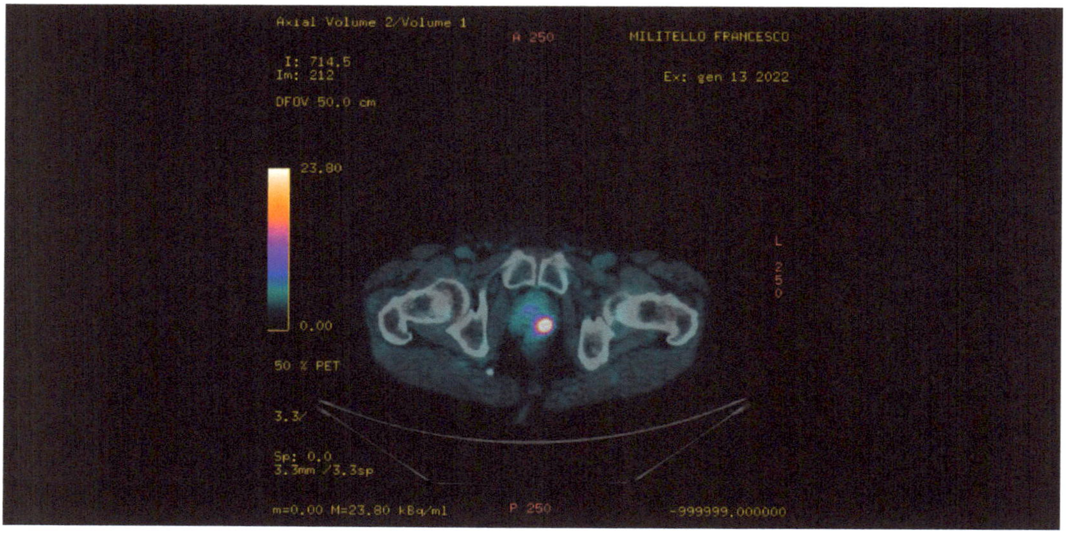

Figure 1. 68Ga-prostate-specific membrane antigen (PSMA) PET/CT: presence of high suspicious area of prostate cancer in the left lobe of prostate gland (axial valuation) with a standardised uptake value (SUVmax) equal to 19.8 g/mL. Targeted biopsy demonstrated the presence of a Grade Group 2 prostate cancer.

All the mpMRI (PI-RADS score > 3) and 68Ga-PET/TC index lesions (SUVmax > 5 g/mL) [15] underwent targeted cores (mpMRI-TPBx and PSMA-TPBx: four cores) combined with saturation prostate biopsy (SPBx: median 20 cores; range 18–22). The procedure was performed transperineally using a tru-cut 18-gauge needle (Bard; Covington, GA, USA) under sedation and antibiotic prophylaxis [16]. The prostate targeted cores were done using an Hitachi 70 Arietta ecograph, Chiba, Japan) supplied by a bi-planar trans-rectal probe [17] performing a free-hand cognitive approach.

3. Results

The clinical parameters of the 30 men enrolled in the active surveillance protocol are listed in Table 1. No selection criteria were used for patients submitted to PET-PSMA evaluation, and no significant differences in terms of clinical parameters were found between these patients and the entire active surveillance group.

Multiparametric MRI and 68Ga-PSMA showed 14/30 (46.6%) and 6/30 (20%) lesions suspicious for PCa those were submitted to targeted cores combined with SPBx. In detail, mpMRI PI-RADS score resulted < 2 vs. 3 vs. 4 in 16 (53.3%) vs. 12 (40%) vs. 2 (6.7%) men. The average intraprostatic SUVmax and tumor dimension was 4.8 g/mL (range: 3.2–19.8) and 7.3 mm (range 4–12 mm), respectively; only 6/30 (20%) men had a SUVmax > 5 g/mL (range: 5.1–19.8 g/mL), moreover, 68Ga-PSMA PET/TC showed two suspicious areas in correspondence of iliac ala and spinal cord; were shown to be negative for metastases in targeted MRI for bone evaluation. In 2/30 (6.6%) men, a csPCa (GG2) was found: both patients had a GPC equal to 20% with a number of positive cores equal to 3 and 4, respectively. PSA density was 0.15 and 0.11.

Table 1. Clinical parameters of 30 men with low-risk prostate cancer (PCa) submitted to scheduled biopsy.

Clinical and Biopsy Findings	GG1 30 Patients
Median PSA (range: 4.5–122 ng/mL)	4.6
Median PSA density (range: 0.10–0.21)	0.15
Median GPC (range: 10–50%)	40%
Median number of positive cores **Percentage of positive cores**	2 9%
mpMRI PI-RADS score ≥ 3	13 (43.3%)
68Ga-PSMA PET/CT suspicious for PCa	6 (20%)

Legend: GG: International Society of Urological Pathology Grade Group; mpMRI: multiparametric magnetic resonance imaging; PSA: prostate-specific antigen; GPC: greatest percentage of cancer; PSMA: Prostate specific membrane antigen; PI-RADS: prostate imaging reporting and data system; PET/TC: positron emission tomography/computed tomography.

68Ga-PSMA-TPBx vs. mpMRI-TPBx vs. SPBx diagnosed 1/2 (50%) vs. 1/2 (50%) vs. 2/2 (100%) csPCa, respectively. In detail, PET/CT PSMA and mpMRI missed the diagnosis of csPCa in two different patients: one patient had a PI-RADS score of 2 and SUVmax of 6.8 g/mL; the man not detected by PSMA PET had a PI-RADS of score 3 at moMRI and SUVmax equal to 4.5 g/mL at 68Ga-PET/TC. In detail, mpMRI and 68Ga-PSMA PET/TC demonstrated 13/30 (43.3%) vs. 5/30 (16.7%) false positive and 1 (50%) vs. 1 (50%) false negative results. In addition, mpMRI and 68Ga-PSMA PET/TC showed a negative predictive value (NPV) in the diagnosis of csPCa equal to 57.1 and 85.7%, respectively.

4. Discussion

The estimated risk-free treatment at 5, 10 and 15 years in men enrolled in AS with GG1 PCa is equal to 76, 64 and 58% [1]; in the last years, many studies have been reported suggesting the best protocol of follow up to reduce the number on scheduled prostate biopsies [1,2]. In this respect, although mpMRI is strongly recommended in the revaluation of men in AS [2,5], scheduled systematic repeated prostate biopsies are still recommended in addition to targeted mpMRI/TRUS fusion biopsy to reduce the false negative rate for csPCa of mpMRI equal to 20% of the cases [17]. At the same time, the number of cores performed at initial repeat evaluation is directly correlated with a lower risk of reclassification [6] during the follow-up, allowing to postpone scheduled repeated prostate biopsy in favour of clinical findings (i.e., PSA density, risk calculator) [18] and imaging revaluation (mpMRI) [5,16,19].

Recently, 68Ga-PSMA-PET/CT has been suggested to improve the clinical stadiation of high-risk PCa and disease recurrence [7]; at the same time, PSMA PET/CT has been proposed for the diagnosis of primary intraprostatic cancer [15]. The presence of focal uptake on PSMA-PET/CT, the standardised uptake value (SUVmax) and the maximal dimensions of PET-avid lesions have been correlated with the presence of csPCa [20,21]. There is a range of proposed cutoffs to detect csPCa from SUVmax 3.15 to up SUVmax 9.1 [22,23]; the concordance between preoperative PSMA PET/TC evaluation (SUVmax, dimension of the lesion), and definitive prostate specimen ranges from 81.2% (24) to 96% [24–28]. Moreover, PSMA PET/MRI seems to reduce the false positive rate of PET/CT (about 3% of cases) [26].

To our knowledge, this is the first study that prospectively evaluated the role of 68Ga- PSMA PET/CT in men enrolled in prostate cancer AS protocols [29]. In our series, 68Ga-PSMA-TPBx vs. mpMRI-TPBx vs. SPBx diagnosed 1/2 (50%) vs. 1/2 (50%) vs. 2/2 (100%) csPCa, respectively. In detail, mpMRI and 68Ga-PSMA PET/TC demonstrated

13/30 (43.3%) vs. 5/30 (16.7%) false positive and 1 (50%) vs. 1 (50%) false negative results. In addition, mpMRI and 68Ga-PSMA PET/TC showed an NPV in in the diagnosis of csPCa equal to 57.1 and 85.7%, respectively.

Diagnostic imaging should not replace scheduled prostate biopsy but is mandatory to detect targeted lesions suspicious for csPCa. Several biochemical parameters, such as thymidine kinase I, mindin or PHI, could be helpful in decrease the ratio of scheduled biopsy. We have no data about these parameters; however, we evaluated our patients according to PSA density, as suggested by latest EAU guidelines.

Among our results, some considerations should be made. First, the number of patients evaluated was low; secondly, the results should be evaluated in the entire prostate specimen and not in biopsy histology. A more detailed histological evaluation of patients who underwent biopsy upstaging would be of interest, for example by adding supplementary staining for PSMA on the biopsy samples. However, this type of staining is not routinely performed at our institution. Third, the low rate of reclassification (6.6% of the cases) could be explained because the patients previously underwent SPBx plus mpMRI evaluation before confirmatory biopsy. Four, 68Ga-PSMA PET/TC evaluation could be proposed in men with negative mpMRI or in the presence of claustrophobia or cardiac pacemaker. Finally, a 68Ga-PSMA PET/TC fusion platform would have increased the accuracy of targeted prostate biopsy.

In conclusion, 68PSMA PET/CT did not improve the detection for csPCa of SPBx (1 false negative result equal to 50% of the cases); at the same time, 68Ga-PSMA PET/CT would have spared 24/30 (80%) scheduled biopsies showing a lower false positive rate in comparison with mpMRI (20% vs. 43.3%) and a better NPV (85.7 vs. 57.1%).

Author Contributions: Conceptualisation, P.P. (Pietro Pepe) and S.C.; methodology, L.P.; investigation, P.P. (Paolo Panella), M.T., G.M., F.S.; data curation, G.C., M.I.; writing—original draft preparation, P.P. (Pietro Pepe), A.T.; writing—review and editing, M.R.; supervision, M.P.; All authors have read and agreed to the published version of the manuscript.

Funding: This research received no external funding.

Institutional Review Board Statement: The study was conducted in accordance with the Declaration of Helsinki, and approved by the Institutional Review Board of Cannizzaro Hospital (protocol code 781/CS date of approval 11th April 2019)" for studies involving humans.

Informed Consent Statement: Informed consent was obtained from all subjects involved in the study.

Data Availability Statement: Data are available at the institutional prostate cancer database of the Urology Unit, Cannizzaro Hospital, Catania.

Conflicts of Interest: Authors declare no conflict of interest.

References

1. Carlsson, S.; Benfante, N.; Alvim, R.; Sjoberg, D.D.; Vickers, A.; Reuter, V.E.; Fine, S.W.; Vargas, H.A.; Wiseman, M.; Mamoor, M.; et al. Long-Term Outcomes of Active Surveillance for Prostate Cancer: The Memorial Sloan Kettering Cancer Center Experience. *J. Urol.* **2020**, *203*, 1122–1127. [CrossRef] [PubMed]
2. Briganti, A.; Fossati, N.; Catto, J.W.; Cornford, P.; Montorsi, F.; Mottet, N.; Wirth, M.; Van Poppel, H. Active Surveillance for Low-risk Prostate Cancer: The European Association of Urology Position in 2018. *Eur. Urol.* **2018**, *74*, 357–368. [CrossRef] [PubMed]
3. Pepe, P.; Cimino, S.; Garufi, A.; Priolo, G.; Russo, G.I.; Giardina, R.; Reale, G.; Pennisi, M.; Morgia, G. Confirmatory biopsy of men under active surveillance: Extended versus saturation versus multiparametric magnetic resonance imaging/transrectal ultrasound fusion prostate biopsy. *Scand. J. Urol.* **2017**, *51*, 260–263. [CrossRef] [PubMed]
4. Pepe, P.; Garufi, A.; Priolo, G.D.; Galia, A.; Fraggetta, F.; Pennisi, M. Is it time to perform only MRI targeted biopsy? Our experi-ence in 1032 men submitted to prostate biopsy. *J. Urol.* **2018**, *200*, 774–778. [CrossRef] [PubMed]
5. Caglic, I.; Sushentsev, N.; Gnanapragasam, V.J.; Sala, E.; Shaida, N.; Koo, B.C.; Kozlov, V.; Warren, A.Y.; Kastner, C.; Barrett, T. MRI-derived PRECISE scores for predicting pathologically-confirmed radiological progression in prostate cancer patients on active surveillance. *Eur. Radiol.* **2021**, *31*, 2696–2705. [CrossRef]

6. Pepe, P.; Pepe, L.; Pennisi, M.; Fraggetta, F. Which Prostate Biopsy in Men Enrolled in Active Surveillance? Experience in 110 Men Submitted to Scheduled Three-Years Transperineal Saturation Biopsy Combined With Fusion Targeted Cores. *Clin. Genitourin. Cancer* **2021**, *19*, 305–308. [CrossRef]
7. Perera, M.; Papa, N.; Roberts, M.; Williams, M.; Udovicich, C.; Vela, I.; Christidis, D.; Bolton, D.; Hofman, M.S.; Lawrentschuk, N.; et al. Gallium-68 prostate-specific membrane antigen positron emission tomography in advanced prostate cancer-updated diagnostic utility, sensitivity, specificity, and distribution of prostate-specific membrane antigen-avid lesions: A systematic review and meta-analysis. *Eur. Urol.* **2020**, *77*, 403–417.
8. Privé, B.M.; Israël, B.; Schilham, M.G.M.; Muselaers, C.H.J.; Zámecnik, P.; Mulders, P.F.A.; Witjes, J.A.; Sedelaar, M.; Mehra, N.; Verzijlbergen, F.; et al. Evaluating F-18-PSMA-1007-PET in primary prostate cancer and comparing it to multi-parametric MRI and histopathology. *Prostate Cancer Prostatic Dis.* **2021**, *24*, 423–430. [CrossRef]
9. Uprimny, C.; Kroiss, A.S.; Decristoforo, C.; Fritz, J.; von Guggenberg, E.; Kendler, D.; Scarpa, L.; Di Santo, G.; Roig, L.G.; Maffey-Steffan, J.; et al. ^{68}Ga-PSMA-11 PET/CT in primary stag-ing of prostate cancer: PSA and Gleason score predict the intensity of tracer accumulation in the primary tumour. *Eur. J. Nucl. Mol. Imaging* **2017**, *44*, 941–949. [CrossRef]
10. Fendler, W.P.; Schmidt, D.F.; Wenter, V.; Thierfelder, K.M.; Zach, C.; Stief, C.; Bartenstein, P.; Kirchner, T.; Gildehaus, F.J.; Gratzke, C.; et al. ^{68}Ga-PSMA PET/CT Detects the Location and Extent of Primary Prostate Cancer. *J. Nucl. Med.* **2016**, *57*, 1720–1725. [CrossRef]
11. Eiber, M.; Weirich, G.; Holzapfel, K.; Souvatzoglou, M.; Haller, B.; Rauscher, I.; Beer, A.J.; Wester, H.-J.; Gschwend, J.; Schwaiger, M.; et al. Simultaneous ^{68}Ga-PSMA HBED-CC PET/MRI Improves the Localization of Primary Prostate Cancer. *Eur. Urol.* **2016**, *70*, 829–836. [CrossRef] [PubMed]
12. Zhang, Q.; Zang, S.; Zhang, C.; Fu, Y.; Lv, X.; Zhang, Q.; Deng, Y.; Zhang, C.; Luo, R.; Zhao, X.; et al. Comparison of ^{68}Ga-PSMA11 PET-CT with mpMRI for preoperative lymph node staging in patients with intermediate to high-risk prostate cancer. *J. Transl. Med.* **2017**, *15*, 230–238. [CrossRef] [PubMed]
13. Raveenthiran, S.; Yaxley, W.J.; Franklin, T.; Coughlin, G.; Roberts, M.; Gianduzzo, T.; Kua, B.; Samaratunga, H.; Delahunt, B.; Egevad, L.; et al. Findings in 1123 Men with Preoperative ^{68}Ga-Prostate-Specific Membrane Antigen Positron Emission Tomography/Computerized Tomography and Multiparametric Magnetic Resonance Imaging Compared to Totally Embedded Radical Prostatectomy Histopathology: Implications for the Diagnosis and Management of Prostate Cancer. *J. Urol.* **2022**, *207*, 573–580. [CrossRef] [PubMed]
14. Epstein, J.I.; Egevad, L.; Amin, M.B.; Delahunt, B.; Srigley, J.R.; Humphrey, P.A.; Grading Committee. The 2014 International Society of Urological Pathology (ISUP) Consensus Conference on Gleason Grading of Prostatic Carcinoma: Definition of Grading Patterns and Proposal for a New Grading System. *Am. J. Surg. Pathol.* **2016**, *40*, 244–252. [CrossRef] [PubMed]
15. Moore, C.M.; Kasivisvanathan, V.; Eggener, S.; Emberton, M.; Fütterer, J.J.; Gill, I.S.; Iii, R.L.G.; Hadaschik, B.; Klotz, L.; Margolis, D.J.; et al. Standards of Reporting for MRI-targeted Biopsy Studies (START) of the Prostate: Recommendations from an International Working Group. *Eur. Urol.* **2013**, *64*, 544–552. [CrossRef]
16. Pepe, P.; Pennisi, M.; Fraggetta, F. How Many Cores Should be Obtained During Saturation Biopsy in the Era of Multiparametric Magnetic Resonance? Experience in 875 Patients Submitted to Repeat Prostate Biopsy. *Urology* **2020**, *137*, 133–137. [CrossRef]
17. Pepe, P.; Garufi, A.; Priolo, G.; Pennisi, M. Can MRI/TRUS fusion targeted biopsy replace saturation prostate biopsy in the re-evaluation of men in active surveillance? *World J. Urol.* **2016**, *34*, 1249–1253. [CrossRef]
18. Roscigno, M.; Stabile, A.; Lughezzani, G.; Pepe, P.; Galosi, A.B.; Naselli, A.; Naspro, R.; Nicolai, M.; La Croce, G.; Aljoulani, M.; et al. The Use of Multiparametric Magnetic Resonance Imaging for Follow-up of Patients Included in Active Surveillance Protocol. Can PSA Density Discriminate Patients at Different Risk of Reclassification? *Clin. Genitourin. Cancer* **2020**, *18*, e698–e704. [CrossRef]
19. Roscigno, M.; Stabile, A.; Lughezzani, G.; Pepe, P.; Dell'Atti, L.; Naselli, A.; Naspro, R.; Nicolai, M.; La Croce, G.; Muhannad, A.; et al. Multiparametric magnetic resonance imaging and clinical variables: Which is the best combination to predict reclassification in active surveillance patients? *Prostate Int.* **2020**, *8*, 167–172. [CrossRef]
20. Kwan, T.N.; Spremo, S.; Teh, A.Y.; McHarg, D.; Thangasamy, I.; Woo, H.H. Performance of Ga-68 PSMA PET/CT for diagnosis and grading of local prostate cancer. *Prostate Int.* **2021**, *9*, 107–112. [CrossRef]
21. Ma, L.; Zhang, W.; Hao, Y. Current state of prostate-specific membrane antigen PET/CT imaging–targeted biopsy techniques for detection of clinically significant prostate cancer. *J. Med. Imaging Radiat. Oncol.* **2021**. [CrossRef] [PubMed]
22. Demirci, E.; Kabasakal, L.; Şahin, O.E.; Akgün, E.; Gültekin, M.H.; Doğanca, T.; Tuna, M.B.; Öbek, C.; Kiliç, M.; Esen, T.; et al. Can SUVmax values of Ga-68-PSMA PET/CT scan predict the clinically significant prostate cancer? *Nucl. Med. Commun.* **2019**, *40*, 86–91. [CrossRef] [PubMed]
23. Rüschoff, J.H.; Ferraro, D.A.; Muehlematter, U.J.; Laudicella, R.; Hermanns, T.; Rodewald, A.K.; Moch, H.; Eberli, D.; Burger, I.A.; Rupp, N.J. What's behind ^{68}Ga-PSMA-11 uptake in primary prostate cancer PET? Investigation of histopathological parameters and immunohisto-chemical PSMA expression patterns. *Eur. J. Nucl. Med. Mol. Imaging* **2021**, *48*, 4042–4053. [CrossRef] [PubMed]
24. Franklin, A.; Yaxley, W.J.; Raveenthiran, S.; Coughlin, G.; Gianduzzo, T.; Kua, B.; McEwan, L.; Wong, D.; Delahunt, B.; Egevad, L.; et al. Histological comparison between predictive value of preoperative 3-T multiparametric MRI and ^{68}Ga-PSMA PET/CT scan for pathological outcomes at radi-cal prostatectomy and pelvic lymph node dissection for prostate cancer. *BJU Int.* **2021**, *127*, 71–79. [CrossRef]

25. Liu, Y.; Yu, H.; Liu, J.; Zhang, X.; Lin, M.; Schmidt, H.; Gao, J.; Xu, B. A Pilot Study of 18F-DCFPyL PET/CT or PET/MRI and Ultrasound Fusion Targeted Prostate Biopsy for Intra-Prostatic PET-Positive Lesions. *Front. Oncol.* **2021**, *11*, 612157. [CrossRef]
26. Kalapara, A.A.; Nzenza, T.; Pan, H.Y.C.; Ballok, Z.; Ramdave, S.; O'Sullivan, R.; Ryan, A.; Cherk, M.; Hofman, M.S.; Konety, B.R.; et al. Detection and localisation of primary prostate cancer using 68 gallium prostate-specific membrane antigen positron emission tomography/computed tomography com-pared with multiparametric magnetic resonance imaging and radical prostatectomy specimen pathology. *BJU Int.* **2020**, *126*, 83–90.
27. Xue, A.L.; Kalapara, A.A.; Ballok, Z.E.; Levy, S.M.; Sivaratnam, D.; Ryan, A.; Ramdave, S.; O'Sullivan, R.; Moon, D.; Grummet, J.P.; et al. ^{68}Ga-Prostate-Specific Membrane Antigen Positron Emission Tomography Maximum Standardized Uptake Value as a Predictor of Gleason Pattern 4 and Pathological Upgrading in Intermediate-Risk Prostate Cancer. *J. Urol.* **2021**, *207*, 341–349. [CrossRef]
28. Zhang, L.L.; Li, W.C.; Xu, Z.; Jiang, N.; Zang, S.M.; Xu, L.W.; Huang, W.B.; Wang, F.; Sun, H.B. ^{68}Ga-PSMA PET/CT targeted biopsy for the diagnosis of clinically significant prostate cancer compared with transrectal ultrasound guided biopsy: A prospective randomized sin-gle-centre study. *Eur. J. Nucl. Med. Mol. Imaging* **2021**, *48*, 483–492. [CrossRef]
29. Bhanji, Y.; Rowe, S.P.; Pavlovich, C.P. New imaging modalities to consider for men with prostate cancer on active surveillance. *World J. Urol.* **2021**, *40*, 51–59. [CrossRef]

Journal of
Clinical Medicine

MDPI

Review

Role of Deep Learning in Prostate Cancer Management: Past, Present and Future Based on a Comprehensive Literature Review

Nithesh Naik [1,2], Theodoros Tokas [3], Dasharathraj K. Shetty [4,*], B.M. Zeeshan Hameed [2,5,*], Sarthak Shastri [6], Milap J. Shah [2,7], Sufyan Ibrahim [2,8], Bhavan Prasad Rai [2,9], Piotr Chłosta [10] and Bhaskar K. Somani [2,11]

1 Department of Mechanical and Industrial Engineering, Manipal Institute of Technology, Manipal Academy of Higher Education, Manipal 576104, Krnataka, India; nithesh.naik@manipal.edu
2 iTRUE (International Training and Research in Uro-Oncology and Endourology) Group, Manipal 576104, Karnataka, India; drmilapshah@gmail.com (M.J.S.); sufyan.ibrahim2@gmail.com (S.I.); urobhavan@gmail.com (B.P.R.); bhaskarsomani@yahoo.com (B.K.S.)
3 Department of Urology and Andrology, General Hospital Hall i.T., Milser Str. 10, 6060 Hall in Tirol, Austria; ttokas@yahoo.com
4 Department of Humanities and Management, Manipal Institute of Technology, Manipal Academy of Higher Education, Manipal 576104, Karnataka, India
5 Department of Urology, Father Muller Medical College, Mangalore 575002, Karnataka, India
6 Department of Information and Communication Technology, Manipal Institute of Technology, Manipal Academy of Higher Education, Manipal 576104, Karnataka, India; sarthak.shastri@learner.manipal.edu
7 Robotics and Urooncology, Max Hospital and Max Institute of Cancer Care, New Delhi 110024, India
8 Kasturba Medical College, Manipal Academy of Higher Education, Manipal 576104, Karnataka, India
9 Department of Urology, Freeman Hospital, Newcastle upon Tyne NE7 7DN, UK
10 Department of Urology, Jagiellonian University in Krakow, Gołębia 24, 31-007 Kraków, Poland; piotr.chlosta@uj.edu.pl
11 Department of Urology, University Hospital Southampton NHS Trust, Southampton SO16 6YD, UK
* Correspondence: raja.shetty@manipal.edu (D.K.S.); zeeshanhameedbm@gmail.com (B.M.Z.H.)

Abstract: This review aims to present the applications of deep learning (DL) in prostate cancer diagnosis and treatment. Computer vision is becoming an increasingly large part of our daily lives due to advancements in technology. These advancements in computational power have allowed more extensive and more complex DL models to be trained on large datasets. Urologists have found these technologies help them in their work, and many such models have been developed to aid in the identification, treatment and surgical practices in prostate cancer. This review will present a systematic outline and summary of these deep learning models and technologies used for prostate cancer management. A literature search was carried out for English language articles over the last two decades from 2000–2021, and present in Scopus, MEDLINE, Clinicaltrials.gov, Science Direct, Web of Science and Google Scholar. A total of 224 articles were identified on the initial search. After screening, 64 articles were identified as related to applications in urology, from which 24 articles were identified to be solely related to the diagnosis and treatment of prostate cancer. The constant improvement in DL models should drive more research focusing on deep learning applications. The focus should be on improving models to the stage where they are ready to be implemented in clinical practice. Future research should prioritize developing models that can train on encrypted images, allowing increased data sharing and accessibility.

Keywords: artificial intelligence; deep learning; convolutional neural network; computer-aided detection; medical imaging; Gleason grading

1. Introduction

Artificial intelligence (AI) is a broad term that incorporates machine learning (ML), in which an algorithm analyzes features in a separate dataset, based on raw input data, without being explicitly programmed, and returns a specific classification [1]. Deep learning (DL) is a subset of ML which uses multilayer artificial neural networks (ANNs) to learn hierarchical representations. Unlike classic ML algorithms such as support vector networks (SVN) and random forest (RF), DL learns features from input data without relying substantially on domain knowledge developed by engineers [2]. Deep learning uses neural networks with many layers where the first layer is the input layer connected to multiple hidden layers that are finally connected to the output layer. Neural networks use a series of algorithms to recognize hidden relationships in a data set by a process similar to the human brain. Each of the interconnected layers comprises numerous nodes, which are called perceptrons. Model perceptrons are arranged to form an interconnected network in a multi-layered perceptron. The input layer, upon receiving the input, transfers patterns obtained to the hidden layers. The hidden layers are activated based on the input parameters received. Hidden layers fine-tune the inputs received until the error is minimal, after which the values of the neurons are passed to the output layer. The activation function calculates the output value, and the neural network produces its result.

Deep learning models help in diagnosing and treating urological conditions and have proved their ability to detect prostate cancer, bladder tumors, renal cell carcinoma, along with ultrasound image analysis. A general schematic diagram of DL models can be seen in Figure 1. Deep learning models have also displayed their ability to detect the needle/trocar pressure during insertion, which is an essential aspect of laparoscopic and robotic urological surgeries.

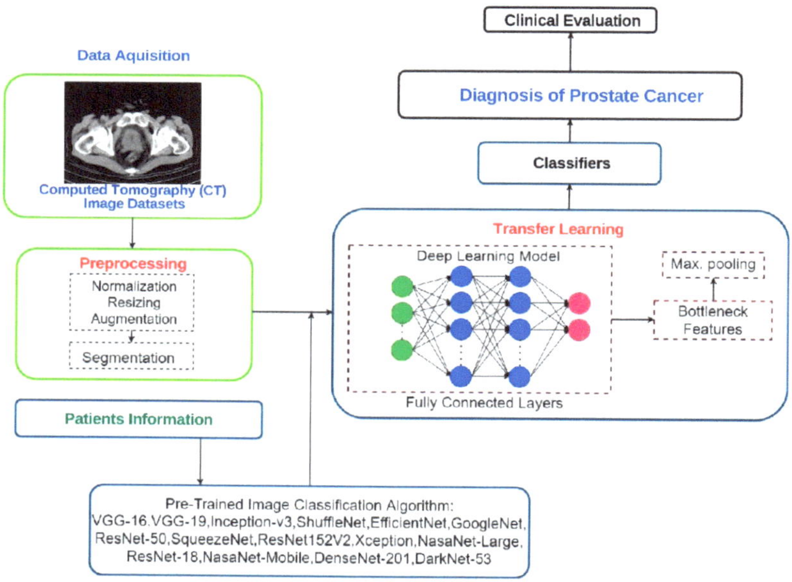

Figure 1. Deep learning framework for image classification.

Supervised learning and unsupervised learning are the two main approaches in AI and machine learning. The primary distinction between the two approaches is the reliance on labelled data in the first, as opposed to the latter. Though the two approaches share many similarities, they also have distinct differences. Figure 2 shows the distinction between the supervised learning and unsupervised learning approach.

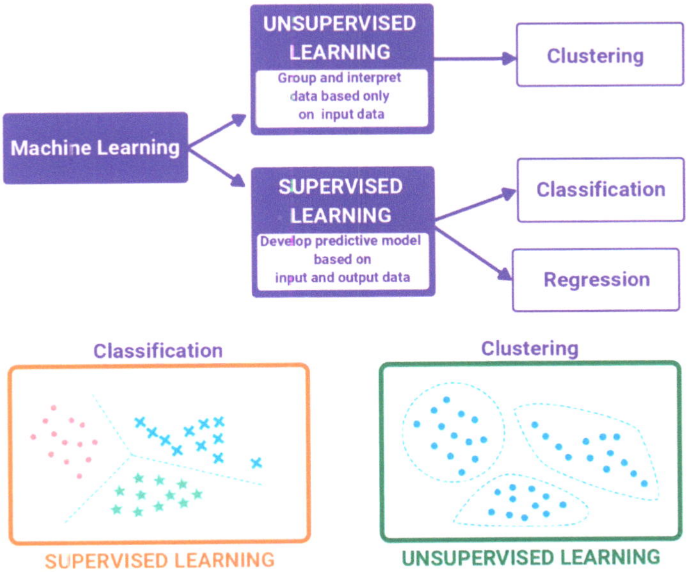

Figure 2. Supervised learning and unsupervised learning approach.

What is supervised learning?

The use of labelled datasets distinguishes supervised learning from other forms of machine learning. Using these datasets, algorithms can be trained to better classify data or predict results. The model's accuracy can be measured and improved over time using labelled inputs and outputs.

Based on data mining, supervised learning can be categorised into two types: classification and regression: (a) classification tasks rely on an algorithm to reliably assign test data to specified groups. For example: supervised learning algorithms can differentiate spam from the rest of the incoming emails. Classification methods include linear classifiers, support vector machines, decision trees, and random forests. (b) Regression is used to learn about the relationship between dependent and independent variables. Predicting numerical values based on various data points is possible with regression models. Linear regression, logistic regression, and polynomial regression are all common regression algorithms.

What is unsupervised learning?

For the analysis and clustering of unlabeled data sets, unsupervised learning makes use of machine learning methods. These algorithms, which are referred to as 'unsupervised', find hidden patterns in data without the aid of human intervention. Three key tasks are performed by unsupervised learning models: (a) clustering, (b) association, and (c) dimensionality reduction.

Using data mining techniques such as clustering, it is possible to create groups of unlabeled data that are similar or dissimilar. Similar data points are grouped together according to the K value in K-means clustering algorithms. This method is useful for a variety of things, including image segmentation and image compression. Another unsupervised learning technique is association, which employs a separate set of criteria to discover connections among the variables in a dataset.

Dimensionality reduction is a learning approach used when the number of features (or dimensions) in a dataset is too large. It minimizes the quantity of data inputs while yet maintaining the integrity of the data. To enhance image quality, auto encoders often utilize this technique to remove noise from visual data before it is processed further.

Over the last decade, imaging technology has significantly improved, which has made it easier for us to apply computer vision technologies for the classification and detection of diseases [3]. With the advancements in graphics processing units (GPUs) and their computational power to perform parallel processing, computer vision processing is more accessible today. Deep learning is also being used for data management, chatbots, and other facilities that aid in medical practice. Natural language processing (NLP) practices used in finding patterns in multimodal data have been shown to increase the learning system's accuracy of diagnosis, prediction, and performance [4]. However, identifying essential clinical elements and establishing relations has been difficult as these records are usually unordered and disorganized. Urology has been at the forefront of accepting newer technologies to achieve better patient outcomes. This comprehensive review aims to give an insight into the applications of deep learning in Urology.

2. Search Strategy

In October 2021, Pubmed/MEDLINE, Scopus, Clinicaltrials.gov, Science Direct, Web of Science and Google Scholar were used to undertake a review of all English language literature published in the previous two decades (2000–2021). The search technique was based on PICO (Patient Intervention Comparison Outcome) criteria, in which patients were treated with AI models (I) or classical biostatistical models (C), and the efficacy of AI models was evaluated (O) [5].

Specifically, the search was conducted by using a combination of the following terms: 'artificial intelligence', 'AI', 'machine learning', 'ML', 'convolutional networks', 'CNN', 'deep learning', 'DL', 'magnetic resonance imaging', 'prostate', 'prostate cancer', 'MRI', 'Sorensen–Dice coefficient', 'DSC', 'area under the ROC curve', 'AUC', 'Sorensen–Dice index', 'SDI' and 'computed tomography', 'CT' [6].

2.1. Inclusion Criteria

1. Articles on the application of deep learning in prostate cancer diagnosis and treatment.
2. Full-text articles, clinical trials and meta-Analysis on outcomes of analysis in Urology using deep learning.

2.2. Exclusion Criteria

1. Animal, laboratory, or cadaveric studies
2. Reviews, editorials, commentaries or book chapters

The literature review was carried out using the inclusion and exclusion criteria mentioned. Articles were screened based on the titles and abstracts. Articles were then selected and their entire text was analyzed. For further screening of other published literature, the references list of the selected articles was individually and manually checked.

3. Results

Evidence Synthesis

A total of 224 distinct articles were discovered during the initial search. Following the initial screening, 97 articles remained, with 64 left after a second screening as related to applications of deep learning in Urology. Among these articles, 24 were identified to be solely related to prostate cancer, these abstracts satisfied our inclusion criteria and were then included in the final review. The summary of all the previous studies from the literature is shown in Tables 1 and 2 on the diagnosis and treatment of prostate cancer, respectively.

Table 1. Summary of studies on diagnosis of prostate cancer using deep learning models.

Author	Year	Objective	Sample Size (n = Patients/Images)	Study Design	Model	AUC	DSC	SDI	MAE	Sn	Sp
A. MRI images											
Takeuchi et al. [7]	2018	To predict PCa using DL and multilayer ANN	334 patients	Prospective	Stepwise ANN 5-hidden-layers	0.76 (Step 200)	N/A	N/A	N/A	N/A	N/A
Schelb et al. [8]	2019	To compare clinical evaluation performance with segmentation-optimized DL system in PCa diagnosis.	312 patients; T2W and diffusion images used	Retrospective	U-Net	N/A	N/A	N/A	N/A	96%	22%
Shao et al. [9]	2021	For PCa diagnosis using ProsRegNet (DL system) using MRI and histopathological data.	152 patients; T2W images and HPE slices used.	Prospective	ProsRegNet and CNNGeometric	N/A	Cohort 1: 0.979 Cohort 2: 0.971 Cohort 3: 0.976	N/A	N/A	N/A	N/A
Hiremath et al. [10]	2021	To detect csPCa using integrated nomogram using DL, PI-RADS grading and clinical factors.	592 patients; T2W and ADC images used	Retrospective	AlexNet and DenseNet	0.76	N/A	N/A	N/A	N/A	N/A
Hiremath et al. [11]	2020	To assess the test-retest repeatability of U-Net (DL system) in identification of csPCa.	112 patients; ADC/DWI images used	Prospective	U-Net	0.8	0.8	N/A	N/A	N/A	N/A
Schelb et al. [12]	2019	The use DL algorithm (U-Net) for detection, localization, and segmentation of csPCa	259 patients; T2W and DW images used.	Retrospective	U-Net	N/A	N/A	N/A	N/A	98%	24%
Yan et al. [13]	2021	For deep combination learning of multi-level features for MR prostate segmentation using a propagation DNN	80 patients; only T2W images used	Retrospective	MatConvNet	N/A	0.84	N/A	N/A	N/A	N/A

Table 1. *Cont.*

Author	Year	Objective	Sample Size (n = Patients/Images)	Study Design	Model	AUC	DSC	SDI	MAE	Sn	Sp
Khosravi et al. [14]	2021	To develop an AI-based model for the early detection of PCa using MR pictures tagged with histopathology information.	400 patients; T2W images used	Retrospective	GoogLenet	0.89	N/A	N/A	N/A	N/A	N/A
Shiradkar et al. [15]	2020	To find any links between T1W and T2W MR fingerprinting data and the appropriate tissue compartment ratios in PCa and prostatitis whole mount histology.	14 patients; T1W and T2 W images used	Retrospective	U-Net	0.997	N/A	N/A	N/A	N/A	N/A
Winkel et al. [16]	2020	To incorporate DL and biparametric imaging for autonomous detection and classification of PI-RADS lesions.	49 patients; T2W and DWI used	Prospective	ProstateAI	N/A	N/A	N/A	N/A	87%	50%
B. Pathology											
AlDubayan et al. [17]	2020	To detect germline harmful mutations in PCa using DL techniques.	1295 patients	Retrospective	Deep Variant and Genome Analysis Toolkit	0.94	N/A	N/A	N/A	CI:0.91–0.97	N/A
Kott et al. [18]	2021	To apply DL methods on biopsy specimen for histopathologic diagnosis and Gleason grading.	85 images 25 patients	Prospective	18-layer CNN	0.83	N/A	N/A	N/A	N/A	N/A
Lucas et al. [19]	2019	To determine Gleason pattern and grade group in biopsy specimen using DL	96 images 38 patients	Retrospective	Inception-v3 CNN	0.92	N/A	N/A	N/A	90%	93%

Table 2. Summary of studies on treatment of prostate cancer using deep learning models.

Author	Year	Objective	Sample Size	Study Design	Model	AUC	DSC	SDI	MAE	Sn	Sp
Sumitomo et al. [20]	2020	To predict risk of urinary incontinence following RARP using DL model based on MRI images	400 patients	Retrospective	CNN model	0.775	N/A	N/A	N/A	N/A	N/A
Lai et al. [21]	2021	To apply DL methods for auto-segmentation of biparametric images into prostate zones and cancer regions.	204 patients; T2W, DWI, ADC images used.	Retrospective	Segnet	0.958	N/A	N/A	N/A	N/A	N/A
Sloun et al. [22]	2020	To use DL for automated real-time prostate segmentation on TRUS pictures.	436 images 181 patients	Prospective	U-Net	0.98	N/A	N/A	N/A	N/A	N/A
Schelb et al. [23]	2020	To compare DL system and multiple radiologists agreement on prostate MRI lesion segmentation	165 patients; T2W and DWI used	Retrospective	U-Net	N/A	0.22	N/A	N/A	N/A	N/A
Soerensen et al. [24]	2021	To develop a DL model for segmenting the prostate on MRI, and apply it in clinics as part of regular MR-US fusion biopsy.	905 patients; T2W images	Prospective	ProGNet and U-Net	N/A	0.92	N/A	N/A	N/A	N/A
Nils et al. [25]	2021	To assess the effects of diverse training data on DL performance in detecting and segmenting csPCa.	1488 images; T2W and DWI images	Retrospective	U-Net	N/A	0.90	N/A	N/A	97%	90%
Polymeri et al. [26]	2019	To validate DL model for automated PCa assessment on PET/CT and evaluation of PET/CT measurements as prognostic indicators	100 patients	Retrospective	Fully CNN	N/A	N/A	0.78	N/A	N/A	N/A
Gentile et al. [27]	2021	To identify high grade PCa using a combination of different PSA molecular forms and PSA density in a DL model.	222 patients	Prospective	7-hidden-layer CNN	N/A	N/A	N/A	N/A	86%	89%
Ma et al. [28]	2017	To autonomously segment CT images using DL and multi-atlas fusion.	92 patients	NA	CNN model	N/A	0.86	N/A	N/A	N/A	N/A
Hung et al. [29]	2019	To develop a DL model to predict urinary continence recovery following RARP and then use it to evaluate the surgeon's past medical results.	79 patients	Prospective	DeepSurv	N/A	N/A	N/A	85.9	N/A	N/A

4. Discussion

4.1. Diagnosis of Prostate Cancer Using MRI Images

Eleven studies have evaluated the application of deep learning in diagnosing prostate cancer.

Takeuchi et al. (2019) developed a DL model to predict prostate cancer using a multi-layer ANN. The model was trained on images obtained from 232 patients and validated its accuracy on images obtained from 102 patients. On a test dataset, the model achieved AUC of 0.76, thereby, suggesting that neural network achieved better results as compared to a logistic regression model. However, this accuracy needs to be improved to be implemented in clinical practice [7].

Khosravi et al. (2021) used DL models to differentiate malignant and benign tumors and high- and low-risk tumors which achieved an AUC of 0.89 and 0.78, respectively. The study concluded that new images captured did not require manual segmentation and could be implemented in clinical practice [14].

Hiremath et al. (2020) used diffusion-weighted imaging fitted with monoexponential function, ADCm, employing a deep learning architecture (U-Net) to investigate the short-term test-retest repeatability of U-Net in slice- and lesion-level identification and segmentation of clinically significant prostate cancer (csPCa: Gleason grade group > 1) (U-Net). The training dataset included 112 PCa patients who had two prostate MRI exams on the same day. Two U-Net-based CNNs were trained using this dataset. The study performed three-fold cross-validation on the training set and evaluated its performance and repeatability on testing data. The CNNs with U-Net-based architecture demonstrated an intraclass correlation coefficient (ICC) between 0.80–0.83, agreement of 66–72%, and DSC of 0.68–0.72 for a slice- and lesion-level detection. These findings lay the groundwork for DL architecture's test-retest and repeatability in identifying and segmenting clinically relevant prostate cancer on apparent diffusion coefficient maps. [11].

To summarize, MR images are most commonly used to study the applications of DL in image-based diagnosis of prostate cancer (PCa). Though the accuracy of the DL models appears to be satisfactory, the generalizability of the results across varied demographics still needs to be tested before implementing into general clinical practice.

4.2. Histopathological Diagnosis of Prostate Cancer Using DL Models

Three studies have evaluated the application of deep learning in the diagnosis of prostate cancer.

Kott et al. (2019) developed a DL algorithm for histopathologic diagnosis. They also performed Gleason grading of the prostate cancer biopsies. This histopathologic diagnosis and Gleason grading process are considered lengthy and time-consuming. Using ML models, this process can be made significantly faster and more efficient. The study was performed using 85 prostate biopsies from 25 patients with further magnification of up to 20x performed. The study used a deep residual CNN model with fivefold cross-validation. The DL model achieved 91.5 and 85.4% accuracy at coarse and fine-level classification, respectively. The study concluded that the model achieved excellent performance for the diagnosis as mentioned earlier; however, it needs to be tested on a larger sample size for external validation [18].

Lucas et al. (2019) performed a study using DL models for automatic Gleason pattern classification to identify grade groups from prostate biopsies. The study used a dataset containing 96 prostate biopsies from 38 patients. The Inception-v3 convolutional neural network was trained to generate probability maps. The model has a 92% accuracy in distinguishing between non-atypical and malignant regions, with a sensitivity and specificity of 90 and 93%, respectively. The study successfully demonstrates the feasibility of training CNN models to differentiate between Gleason patterns in heterogeneous biopsies [19].

The DL models have shown promising results in the histopathological diagnosis of PCa. This can definitely be added as an adjunct tool for the histopathologists to reduce the burden in terms of time and workload. However due to lack of external validation of these models, their applicability cannot be generalized as of yet.

4.3. Diagnosis of Prostate Cancer Using MR Based Segmentation Techniques

Four studies have evaluated the application of DL in the diagnosis of prostate cancer.

Lai et al. (2021) developed a DL CNN model to segment prostate zones and cancer regions from MRI images. The study was performed using the PROSTATEx dataset containing MRI scans from 204 patients. A SegNet model was modified and fine-tuned to perform adequately on the dataset. The study achieved a dice similarity coefficient of 90.45% for the transition zone, 70.04% for the peripheral zone, and 52.73% for the prostate cancer region. The study concluded that automatic segmentation using a DCNN model has the potential to assist in prostate cancer diagnosis [21].

Sloun et al. (2021) performed prostate segmentation of transrectal ultrasound using the DL model on MRI images. The study used three datasets with MRI-transrectal ultrasound images collected at different institutions. The study trained a U-Net model on the dataset of 436 images and achieved a median accuracy of 98%. While performing zonal segmentation, the model achieved a pixel-wise accuracy of 97 and 98% for the peripheral and transition images. The model can also self-assess its segmentation, allowing it to identify incorrect segmentations swiftly. The process of performing manual segmentation of prostate MRI images places a burden on clinicians. The authors concluded that using DL models can allow for fast and accurate segmentation of MRI images from different scanners [22].

Schelb et al. (2020) produced a comparison of prostate MRI lesion segmentation between a DL model and multiple radiologists. The study was performed using MRI images collected from 165 patients suspected to have prostate cancer. The study used U-Net models trained on the dataset of MRI images to perform segmentation. The mean Dice coefficient for manual segmentation was between 0.48–0.52, while the U-Net segmentations exhibited a Dice coefficient of 0.22. The authors concluded that smaller segmentation sizes could explain the lower Dice coefficients of the U-Net model. They also discuss how the overlapping lesions between multiple rates can be used as a secondary measure for segmentation quality in future studies [23].

Soerensen et al. (2021) performed a study to determine if DL improves the speed and accuracy of prostate gland segmentation from MRI images. The study used images from 905 subjects who underwent prostate MRI scans at 29 institutions. The study trained a ProGNet model on 805 cases and tested it on 100 independent and 56 external cases. The study found that the ProGNet model outperformed the U-Net model. The study also found that the ProGNet model achieved a Dice similarity coefficient of 0.93, outperforming radiology technicians, producing results at 35 s/case. The study concluded that DL models could be used for segmentation in targeted biopsy in routine urological clinical practice [24].

As proven, ProGNet model outperformed not only the U-Net model but also the radiology technicians in terms of speed and accuracy. However, it should be noted that authors have not compared the ProGNet model to trained and experienced urologists and radiologists. Furthermore, the accuracy of the model has to be tested across different MRI scanners.

4.4. Diagnosis of Prostate Cancer Using CT Images

Four studies have evaluated the application of DL in the diagnosis of prostate cancer and prostatectomy. Polymeri et al. (2019) used a DL algorithm to automate prostate cancer quantification on positron emission tomography–computed tomography (PET/CT) scans. The study looked at the possibility of PET/CT measurements as prognostic biomarkers. The training of the DL model was performed on CT scan images of 100 patients. In 45 patients with biopsy-proven hormone-naive prostate cancer, the DL algorithm was validated. The model was evaluated based on the Sørensen–Dice index (SDI) score. The SDI scores achieved were 0.78 and 0.79 for automatic and manual volume segmentation, respectively. The study demonstrated DL applications in quantifying PET/CT prostate gland uptake and its association with overall survival. The results obtained showed agreement between automated and manual PET/CT measurements. The DL model demonstrated that PET/CT indicators were strongly linked to overall survival [26].

Ma et al. (2017) performed automatic prostate segmentation using DL and multi-atlas fusion. A dataset of 92 prostate CT scans was used to conduct and assess the study. When compared to the radiologists' manual segmentation, the model had a Dice similarity coefficient of 86.80%. The study concluded that the DL-based method can provide a valuable tool for automatic segmentation and aid clinical practice [28].

Not many studies have been performed to check the applications of DL models using PET/CT images to highlight their advantages in the same aspect. However, the nascent applications appear promising in terms of development of DL-based biomarker and prognostic models.

4.5. Robot-Assisted Treatment Practices

The study by Hung et al. evaluated the application of DL in the treatment of PCa and RARP. Hung et al. created a DL model to predict urinary continence recovery following radical prostatectomy with robotic assistance. The study was performed on images obtained from 79 patients. The study trained a DeepSurv model on the dataset and achieved a concordance index (C-index) of 0.6 and a mean absolute error (MAE) of 85.9 in predicting continence. The authors concluded that using automated performance metrics and clinicopathological data, the DeepSurv model could predict continence after the prostatectomy. According to the findings, experienced surgeons had greater continence rates at 3 and 6 months following the prostatectomy [29].

The application of automated performance metrics (APMs) and its impact on clinical outcome variables was very well highlighted in this study, underlining the evidence that surgical skills impact clinical outcomes. However, this was a single-institution study and requires external validation for the same.

4.6. Strengths, limitations, and Areas of Future Research

A wide variety of DL models were used to diagnose and treat prostate cancer. The review contains various implementations of DL which benefit the urologists. A summary of the various models used can be viewed in the table as shown (Table 3). One of the major drawbacks of the present study is the small dataset and lack of federated learning approach. Federated learning models can be implemented to improve the data collection and sharing process for research purposes. Increasing the sample size may improve the performance of multilayer DL models as a result of more sufficient training. If the sample size is increased, neural networks with more hidden layers and nodes can perform better, avoiding early over-fitting. An increase in the variables used for prostate cancer detection can also augment the performance of a neural network model. With advanced DL models such as the single shot detector model, it is possible to make predictions on a live video feed during treatment. The live feed DL models can also program robots to help during surgeries.

Table 3. Summary of common deep learning models used in PCa management.

Diagnosis Using MRI Images	Diagnosis Using CT Images	Treatment Using MRI Images	Treatment Using CT Images
DenseNet	NiftyNet	SegNet	7-Hidden Layer CNN
U-Net	InceptionV3		U-Net
AlexNet	Stepwise Neural Network with five hidden layers	U-Net	ProgNet
MatConvNet	18-layer CNN		

5. Conclusions

As per our review, the most common application of DL techniques has been in the diagnosis of prostate cancer using MR image-based segmentation techniques. Although the ProgNet model outperformed trained radiologists in prostate cancer detection, we cannot generalize these results. In conclusion, for clinical application, the DL models' performance may still need improvement. As the performance of these models increases, they will become much more implementable, with many models surpassing human accuracy and efficiency.

Author Contributions: Concept and Study design: B.M.Z.H., B.K.S., T.T., N.N. and B.P.R.; Methods and experimental work: T.T., S.S., M.J.S. and P.C.; Results analysis and conclusions: B.M.Z.H., B.K.S., N.N., S.I and B.P.R.; Manuscript preparation: N.N., S.S., S.I., M.J.S. and D.K.S. All authors have read and agreed to the published version of the manuscript.

Funding: This research received no specific grant from any funding agency in the public, commercial, or not-for-profit sectors.

Institutional Review Board Statement: Not applicable.

Informed Consent Statement: Not applicable.

Data Availability Statement: Not applicable.

Conflicts of Interest: The authors declare no conflict of interest.

References

1. Pannala, R.; Krishnan, K.; Melson, J.; Parsi, M.A.; Schulman, A.R.; Sullivan, S.; Trikudanathan, G.; Trindade, A.J.; Watson, R.R.; Maple, J.T.; et al. Artificial intelligence in gastrointestinal endoscopy. *VideoGIE* **2020**, *5*, 598–613. [CrossRef]
2. Chen, H.; Sung, J. Potentials of AI in medical image analysis in Gastroenterology and Hepatology. *J. Gastroenterol. Hepatol.* **2021**, *36*, 31–38. [CrossRef] [PubMed]
3. Ganatra, N.; Patel, A. A comprehensive study of deep learning architectures, applications and tools. *Int. J. Comput. Sci. Eng.* **2018**, *6*, 701–705. [CrossRef]
4. Asgari, S.; Scalzo, F.; Kasprowicz, M. Pattern recognition in medical decision support. *BioMed Res. Int.* **2019**, *2019*, 2. [CrossRef] [PubMed]
5. Eriksen, M.; Frandsen, T. The impact of patient, intervention, comparison, outcome (PICO) as a search strategy tool on literature search quality: A systematic review. *J. Med. Libr. Assoc.* **2018**, *106*, 420–431. [CrossRef] [PubMed]
6. Liberati, A.; Altman, D.G.; Tetzlaff, J.; Mulrow, C.; Gøtzsche, P.C.; Ioannidis, J.P.; Clarke, M.; Devereaux, P.J.; Kleijnen, J.; Moher, D. The PRISMA statement for reporting systematic reviews and meta-analyses of studies that evaluate healthcare interventions: Explanation and elaboration. *BMJ* **2009**, *339*, b2700. [CrossRef] [PubMed]
7. Takeuchi, T.; Hattori-Kato, M.; Okuno, Y.; Iwai, S.; Mikami, K. Prediction of prostate cancer by deep learning with multilayer artificial neural network. *Can. Urol. Assoc. J.* **2018**, *13*, E145–E150. [CrossRef] [PubMed]
8. Schelb, P.; Kohl, S.; Radtke, J.P.; Wiesenfarth, M.; Kickingereder, P.V.; Bickelhaupt, S.; Kuder, T.A.; Stenzinger, A.; Hohenfellner, M.; Schlemmer, H.-P.; et al. Classification of cancer at prostate MRI: Deep learning versus clinical PI-RADS assessment. *Radiology* **2019**, *293*, 607–617. [CrossRef]
9. Shao, W.; Banh, L.; Kunder, C.A.; Fan, R.E.; Soerensen, S.J.; Wang, J.B.; Teslovich, N.C.; Madhuripan, N.; Jawahar, A.; Ghanouni, P.; et al. ProsRegNet: A deep learning framework for registration of MRI and histopathology images of the prostate. *Med. Image Anal.* **2021**, *68*, 101919. [CrossRef]
10. Hiremath, A.; Shiradkar, R.; Fu, P.; Mahran, A.; Rastinehad, A.R.; Tewari, A.; Tirumani, S.H.; Purysko, A.; Ponsky, L.; Madabhushi, A. An integrated nomogram combining deep learning, Prostate Imaging-Reporting and Data System (PI-RADS) scoring, and clinical variables for identification of clinically significant prostate cancer on biparametric MRI: A retrospective multicentre study. *Lancet Digit. Health* **2021**, *3*, e445–e454. [CrossRef]
11. Hiremath, A.; Shiradkar, R.; Merisaari, H.; Prasanna, P.; Ettala, O.; Taimen, P.; Aronen, H.J.; Boström, P.J.; Jambor, I.; Madabhushi, A. Test-retest repeatability of a deep learning architecture in detecting and segmenting clinically significant prostate cancer on apparent diffusion coefficient (ADC) maps. *Eur. Radiol.* **2020**, *31*, 379–391. [CrossRef] [PubMed]
12. Schelb, P.; Wang, X.; Radtke, J.P.; Wiesenfarth, M.; Kickingereder, P.; Stenzinger, A.; Hohenfellner, M.; Schlemmer, H.-P.; Maier-Hein, K.H.; Bonekamp, D. Simulated clinical deployment of fully automatic deep learning for clinical prostate MRI assessment. *Eur. Radiol.* **2021**, *31*, 302–313. [CrossRef] [PubMed]
13. Yan, Y.; Shao, L.; Liu, Z.; He, W.; Yang, G.; Liu, J.; Xia, H.; Zhang, Y.; Chen, H.; Liu, C.; et al. Deep learning with quantitative features of magnetic resonance images to predict biochemical recurrence of radical prostatectomy: A multi-center study. *Cancers* **2021**, *13*, 3098. [CrossRef] [PubMed]

14. Khosravi, P.; Lysandrou, M.; Eljalby, M.; Li, Q.; Kazemi, E.; Zisimopoulos, P.; Sigaras, A.; Brendel, M.; Barnes, J.; Ricketts, C.; et al. A deep learning approach to diagnostic classification of prostate cancer using pathology-radiology fusion. *J. Magn. Reson. Imaging* **2021**, *54*, 462–471. [CrossRef] [PubMed]
15. Shiradkar, R.; Panda, A.; Leo, P.; Janowczyk, A.; Farre, X.; Janaki, N.; Li, L.; Pahwa, S.; Mahran, A.; Buzzy, C.; et al. T1 and T2 MR fingerprinting measurements of prostate cancer and prostatitis correlate with deep learning–derived estimates of epithelium, lumen, and stromal composition on corresponding whole mount histopathology. *Eur. Radiol.* **2020**, *31*, 1336–1346. [CrossRef] [PubMed]
16. Winkel, D.J.; Wetterauer, C.; Matthias, M.O.; Lou, B.; Shi, B.; Kamen, A.; Comaniciu, D.; Seifert, H.-H.; Rentsch, C.A.; Boll, D.T. Autonomous detection and classification of PI-RADS lesions in an MRI screening population incorporating multicenter-labeled deep learning and biparametric imaging: Proof of concept. *Diagnostics* **2020**, *10*, 951. [CrossRef]
17. Aldubayan, S.H.; Conway, J.R.; Camp, S.Y.; Witkowski, L.; Kofman, E.; Reardon, B.; Han, S.; Moore, N.; Elmarakeby, H.; Salari, K.; et al. Detection of pathogenic variants with germline genetic testing using deep learning vs standard methods in patients with prostate cancer and melanoma. *JAMA* **2020**, *324*, 1957. [CrossRef]
18. Kott, O.; Linsley, D.; Amin, A.; Karagounis, A.; Jeffers, C.; Golijanin, D.; Serre, T.; Gershman, B. Development of a deep learning algorithm for the histopathologic diagnosis and gleason grading of prostate cancer biopsies: A pilot study. *Eur. Urol. Focus* **2021**, *7*, 347–351. [CrossRef]
19. Lucas, M.; Jansen, I.; Savci-Heijink, C.D.; Meijer, S.L.; de Boer, O.J.; van Leeuwen, T.G.; de Bruin, D.M.; Marquering, H.A. Deep learning for automatic Gleason pattern classification for grade group determination of prostate biopsies. *Virchows Arch.* **2019**, *475*, 77–83. [CrossRef]
20. Sumitomo, M.; Teramoto, A.; Toda, R.; Fukami, N.; Fukaya, K.; Zennami, K.; Ichino, M.; Takahara, K.; Kusaka, M.; Shiroki, R. Deep learning using preoperative magnetic resonance imaging information to predict early recovery of urinary continence after robot-assisted radical prostatectomy. *Int. J. Urol.* **2020**, *27*, 922–928. [CrossRef]
21. Lai, C.-C.; Wang, H.-K.; Wang, F.-N.; Peng, Y.-C.; Lin, T.-P.; Peng, H.-H.; Shen, S.-H. Autosegmentation of prostate zones and cancer regions from biparametric magnetic resonance images by using deep-learning-based neural networks. *Sensors* **2021**, *21*, 2709. [CrossRef] [PubMed]
22. Van Sloun, R.J.; Wildeboer, R.R.; Mannaerts, C.K.; Postema, A.W.; Gayet, M.; Beerlage, H.P.; Salomon, G.; Wijkstra, H.; Mischi, M. Deep learning for real-time, automatic, and scanner-adapted prostate (zone) segmentation of transrectal ultrasound, for example, magnetic resonance imaging–transrectal ultrasound fusion prostate biopsy. *Eur. Urol. Focus* **2021**, *7*, 78–85. [CrossRef] [PubMed]
23. Schelb, P.; Tavakoli, A.A.; Tubtawee, T.; Hielscher, T.; Radtke, J.-P.; Görtz, M.; Schütz, V.; Kuder, T.A.; Schimmöller, L.; Stenzinger, A.; et al. Comparison of prostate MRI lesion segmentation agreement between multiple radiologists and a fully automatic deep learning system. *RöFo—Fortschr. Geb. Röntgenstrahlen Bildgeb. Verfahr.* **2020**, *193*, 559–573. [CrossRef] [PubMed]
24. Soerensen, S.J.C.; Fan, R.E.; Seetharaman, A.; Chen, L.; Shao, W.; Bhattacharya, I.; Kim, Y.H.; Sood, R.; Borre, M.; Chung, B.I.; et al. Deep learning improves speed and accuracy of prostate gland segmentations on magnetic resonance imaging for targeted biopsy. *J. Urol.* **2021**, *206*, 604–612. [CrossRef] [PubMed]
25. Netzer, N.; Weißer, C.; Schelb, P.; Wang, X.; Qin, X.; Görtz, M.; Schütz, V.; Radtke, J.P.; Hielscher, T.; Schwab, C.; et al. Fully automatic deep learning in bi-institutional prostate magnetic resonance imaging: Effects of cohort size and heterogeneity. *Investig. Radiol.* **2021**, *56*, 799–808. [CrossRef] [PubMed]
26. Polymeri, E.; Sadik, M.; Kaboteh, R.; Borrelli, P.; Enqvist, O.; Ulén, J.; Ohlsson, M.; Trägårdh, E.; Poulsen, M.H.; Simonsen, J.A.; et al. Deep learning-based quantification of PET/CT prostate gland uptake: Association with overall survival. *Clin. Physiol. Funct. Imaging* **2019**, *40*, 106–113. [CrossRef]
27. Gentile, F.; Ferro, M.; Della Ventura, B.; La Civita, E.; Liotti, A.; Cennamo, M.; Bruzzese, D.; Velotta, R.; Terracciano, D. Optimised identification of high-grade prostate cancer by combining different PSA molecular forms and PSA density in a deep learning model. *Diagnostics* **2021**, *11*, 335. [CrossRef]
28. Ma, L.; Guo, R.; Zhang, G.; Tade, F.; Schuster, D.M.; Nieh, P.; Master, V.; Fei, B. Automatic segmentation of the prostate on CT images using deep learning and multi-atlas fusion. *Med. Imaging* **2017**, *10133*, 101332O.
29. Hung, A.J.; Chen, J.; Ghodoussipour, S.; Oh, P.J.; Liu, Z.; Nguyen, J.; Purushotham, S.; Gill, I.S.; Liu, Y. A deep-learning model using automated performance metrics and clinical features to predict urinary continence recovery after robot-assisted radical prostatectomy. *BJU Int.* **2019**, *124*, 487–495. [CrossRef]

Journal of
Clinical Medicine

MDPI

Article

Radiomics in PI-RADS 3 Multiparametric MRI for Prostate Cancer Identification: Literature Models Re-Implementation and Proposal of a Clinical–Radiological Model

Andrea Corsi [1,2,*,†], Elisabetta De Bernardi [3,4,†], Pietro Andrea Bonaffini [1,2], Paolo Niccolò Franco [1,2], Dario Nicoletta [1,2], Roberto Simonini [1,2], Davide Ippolito [2,5], Giovanna Perugini [1], Mariaelena Occhipinti [6], Luigi Filippo Da Pozzo [2,7], Marco Roscigno [2,7] and Sandro Sironi [1,2]

1 Department of Radiology, ASST Papa Giovanni XXIII, Piazza OMS 1, 24127 Bergamo, Italy
2 School of Medicine, University of Milano-Bicocca, Piazza dell'Ateneo Nuovo 1, 20126 Milan, Italy
3 Medicine and Surgery Department, University of Milano-Bicocca, Via Cadore 48, 20900 Monza, Italy
4 Interdepartmental Research Centre Bicocca Bioinformatics Biostatistics and Bioimaging Centre-B4, University of Milano-Bicocca, Via Follereau 3, 20854 Vedano al Lambro, Italy
5 Department of Radiology, San Gerardo Hospital, Via G. B. Pergolesi 33, 20900 Monza, Italy
6 Radiomics, Boulevard Patience et Beaujonc 3, 4000 Liège, Belgium
7 Department of Urology, ASST Papa Giovanni XXIII, Piazza OMS 1, 24127 Bergamo, Italy
* Correspondence: dr.andreacorsi@gmail.com; Tel.: +39-393-426-8216
† These authors contributed equally to this work.

Abstract: PI-RADS 3 prostate lesions clinical management is still debated, with high variability among different centers. Identifying clinically significant tumors among PI-RADS 3 is crucial. Radiomics applied to multiparametric MR (mpMR) seems promising. Nevertheless, reproducibility assessment by external validation is required. We retrospectively included all patients with at least one PI-RADS 3 lesion (PI-RADS v2.1) detected on a 3T prostate MRI scan at our Institution (June 2016–March 2021). An MRI-targeted biopsy was used as ground truth. We assessed reproducible mpMRI radiomic features found in the literature. Then, we proposed a new model combining PSA density and two radiomic features (texture regularity (T2) and size zone heterogeneity (ADC)). All models were trained/assessed through 100-repetitions 5-fold cross-validation. Eighty patients were included (26 with GS $\geq$ 7). In total, 9/20 T2 features (Hector's model) and 1 T2 feature (Jin's model) significantly correlated to biopsy on our dataset. PSA density alone predicted clinically significant tumors (sensitivity: 66%; specificity: 71%). Our model obtained a sensitivity of 80% and a specificity of 76%. Standard-compliant works with detailed methodologies achieve comparable radiomic feature sets. Therefore, efforts to facilitate reproducibility are needed, while complex models and imaging protocols seem not, since our model combining PSA density and two radiomic features from routinely performed sequences appeared to differentiate clinically significant cancers.

Keywords: PI-RADS 3; prostate cancer; MRI; radiomics; texture analysis

1. Introduction

Prostate cancer (PC) is the second leading tumor in the male population worldwide [1]. Multiparametric magnetic resonance imaging (mpMRI) is the gold standard for prostate cancer imaging nowadays, proven to be helpful in early diagnosis, being employed in the evaluation of prostate gland lesions, local T-staging or recurrence, and in the assessment of pelvic lymph nodes involvement [2] along with Prostate Imaging Reporting and Data System version 2.1 (PI-RADS v2.1) guidelines [3]. Many studies have demonstrated a high correlation between PI-RADS and the Gleason score (GS) of prostate lesions [4–7]. However, while PI-RADS 4/5 are considered highly suspicious for neoplasia, the presence of clinically significant cancer in PI-RADS 3 lesions is equivocal (16–21% reported prevalence) [8,9]. Consequently, there is no consensus on the clinical management of PI-RADS 3 lesions, with high variability in protocols used in different centers [10]. A prostate biopsy is mandatory for diagnosis, but it is associated with possible complications (prostatitis, urinary tract infections, and sepsis), which may lead to hospitalization and, in the worst cases, even death. Therefore, it is crucial to timely identify clinically significant tumors (i.e., lesions with a Gleason Score (GS) ≥ 7, according to current literature [11]) among PI-RADS 3 lesions [12,13].

Some single-center studies in the literature have tried to exploit mpMRI radiomic analysis to identify clinically significant prostate cancer (csPCa) with promising results [14–19]. However, each center found its own radiomic features pool, likely due to high variability in center-specific population features, gold-standard definition rules, scanners, acquisition parameters, lesion contouring, image preprocessing, and machine learning techniques [20,21]. Furthermore, single-center datasets are almost always unavoidably small, increasing the risk of scarcely robust internal validation. Two papers on PI-RADS 3–5 recently showed that single-center models have a significant performance drop when applied to other centers' data [22,23]. Efforts must therefore be made to (1) standardize as much as possible (as in radiomic features computation) [24]; (2) build large and multi-center datasets; (3) share developed models for external validation. This will allow us to understand whether general models can work even with center-specific variabilities or if center-specific models are needed instead.

On this basis, the aim of this work is manifold as follows: (a) to assess reproducible csPCa identification models found in the literature on an independent 80-patient dataset while providing details on their architectures; (b) to propose a new csPCa identification model for external validation based on robustly selected and easily obtainable radiomic and clinical features.

2. Materials and Methods

2.1. Study Population

We retrospectively retrieved medical and radiological data from our Institution's Electronic Medical Records. According to urological indication, the initial population included 945 males who underwent prostate MRI (June 2016–March 2021) for suspected malignancy or active surveillance. From the original cohort, 706 patients were excluded for the following: (a) lack of one/more PI-RADS 3 lesion(s) as per PI-RADS v2.1 (n = 691); (b) no histopathological data within twelve months from MRI scan (n = 11); (c) poor image quality of diffusion-weighted (DWI) and/or in the T2-weighted sequences (n = 2) and apparent diffusion coefficient (ADC) map (n = 1). Accordingly, the final cohort included 80 males.

We collected the following clinical and laboratoristic data (Table 1): age, the most recent serological value of prostate-specific antigen (PSA; ng/mL), PSA density (total PSA/prostatic volume ratio), final histopathological analysis, and mean ADC value (mm^2/s) calculated in a single 2D region of interest (ROI), i.e., the largest trackable circular area in the center of the lesion without exceeding the lesion margins.

2.2. MR Protocol and PI-RADS 3 Lesion Selection

Prostate MRIs were performed on a 3T scanner (Discovery MR750w GEM, GE Healthcare, Chicago, IL, USA), using a 16-channels pelvic anterior-array coil (GE Healthcare, Chicago, IL, USA), and with the patient supine. As per PI-RADS v2.1 criteria [3], MRIs were performed at least six weeks after any prostatic biopsy to avoid a possible source of diagnostic errors due to post-procedural bleeding foci. The standard MRI protocol is summarized in Table 2.

Blinded to pathological data, two radiology residents (A.C., P.N.F.; 3 years of experience) reviewed all MRIs in consensus, based on the current standard of care, considering the appearance of the lesions in the T2-w, DWI, ADC, and DCE sequences as per PI-RADS v2.1 [3]. For each patient, we selected a single target lesion (the largest one in case of multiple lesions). A board-certified radiologist (P.A.B.; 10 years of experience) validated the selection.

Table 1. Characteristics of the final study population.

Population Data	
Total, n	80
Age (years), average ± SD (range)	65.2 ± 7.6 (45–81)
PSA (ng/mL), average ± SD (range)	6.8 ± 4.8 (0.5–29.6)
PSA Density, average ± SD (range)	0.15 ± 0.15 (0.01–1.09)
Mean ADC value within 2D ROI (mm^2/s)	0.000825 ± 0.000253 (0.00026–0.00141)
PI-RADS 3 lesions histology, n/total (%)	
GS ≥ 3 + 4	26/80 (32.5%)
GS ≤ 3 + 3	16/80 (20.0%)
Negative, BPH, atrophy	38/80 (47.5%)
Site of PI-RADS 3 lesions, n/total (%)	
Transitional zone	14/80 (17.5%)
Peripheral zone	66/80 (82.5%)

PSA: prostate-specific antigen; PSA density is obtained by dividing PSA levels (ng/mL) by the volume of the prostatic gland (mL); PI-RADS: Prostate Imaging-Reporting and Data System; BPH: benign prostatic hyperplasia.

Table 2. MRI acquisition parameters.

	T1-w		T2-w		DWI
Acquisition plane	Axial	Axial	Axial, coronal, sagittal	Axial	Axial
Sequence	Fast spin-echo (SSFSE)	Gradient-recalled echo (GRE); before and after intravenous contrast (DCE)	Fast relaxation fast spin echo (FR-FSE)	Single-shot fast spin echo (SS-FSE)	b values: 50, 1000, 2000 s/mm^2
Slice thickness	4 mm	3 mm	3 mm	4 mm	3 mm
Covered area	Pelvis	Prostate lodge and seminal vesicles	Prostate lodge and seminal vesicles	Pelvis	Prostate lodge

DWI: diffusion-weighted imaging; GRE: gradient-recalled echo; DCE: dynamic contrast enhancement; FRFSE: fast relaxation fast spin echo; SSFSE: single-shot fast spin echo.

2.3. Pathological Examination

Each patient underwent a targeted biopsy of PI-RADS 3 lesions (4 cores) at our Institution. Biopsies were executed by a single operator with a total experience of more than 500 target fusion biopsies. We used the trans-rectal access and fusion technique with the reference MRI, a MyLabClassC ultrasound machine, and a virtual navigator fusion system (Esaote S.p.A., Genova, Italy) equipped with an end-fire endorectal probe. Additional systematic biopsies (12–16 cores, according to the following prostate volume: ≤60 mL vs. >60 mL) were performed (Figures 1 and 2) [25]. It was thus possible to choose the prostate parenchymal tissue corresponding to the PI-RADS 3 target lesion as the reference standard. Gleason Score was assigned per 2005 ISUP recommendations (International Society of Urological Pathology) [26]. Each PCa-positive biopsy was evaluated according to the International Society of Urological Pathology 2014 consensus Gleason Grade Group system [11].

2.4. Lesion Segmentation

Anonymized DICOM files of FRFSE-T2-weighted sequences, DWI 2000 s/mm^2 sequences, and ADC maps were exported and loaded on dedicated segmentation software, ITK-SNAP 3.8.0 (PICSL, University of Pennsylvania, Philadelphia, PA, USA) [27]. The 3D ROIs were manually delineated on every target lesion (Figure 3), both on T2-weighted sequences and DWI sequences/ADC maps in consensus by two radiology residents (A.C. and P.N.F.; 3 years of experience), and then validated by a board-certified radiologist (P.A.B.; 10 years of experience). Peripheral zone lesions were visible on both T2-weighted and DWI sequences/ADC maps. When a transitional zone lesion was not readily discernible on DWI/ADC maps, the segmentation area was delineated according to that traced on the T2-weighted sequence. An additional 3D ROI for each patient was outlined in the peripheral prostate zone to normalize intensity, avoiding potential focal lesions. Images were all corrected for magnetic field inhomogeneity (algorithm N4, 3D Slicer, http://www.slicer.org (accessed on 17 September 2022)).

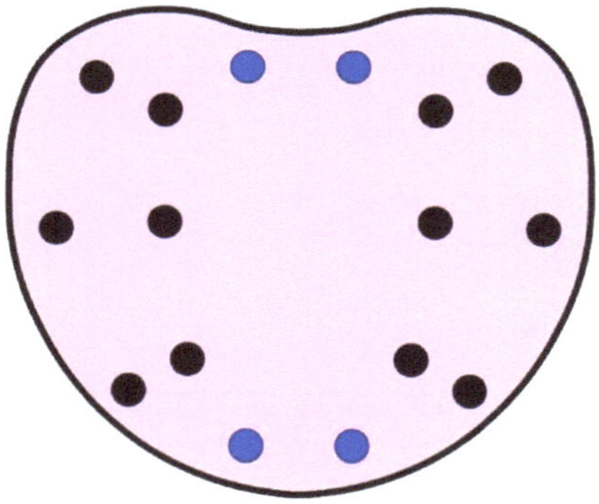

Figure 1. Scheme of systematic template for prostate biopsy. Black dots represent systematic biopsies. Blue dots represent additional systematic biopsies according to prostate volume (>60 mL).

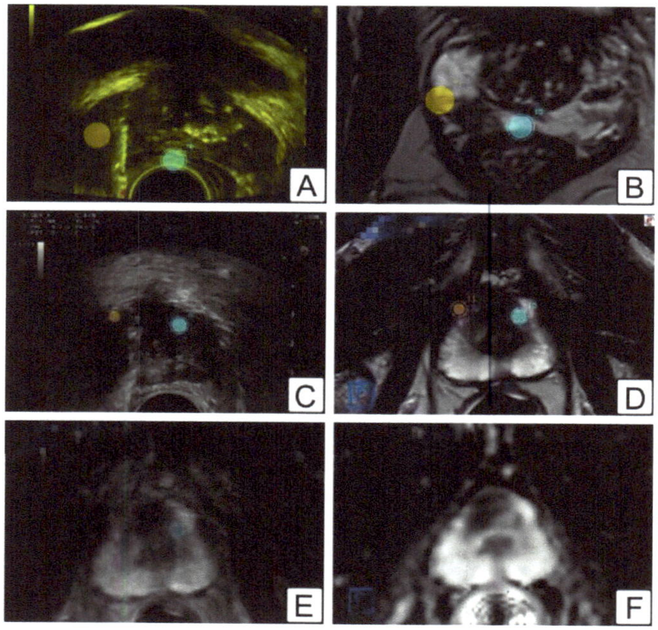

Figure 2. Illustrations of MRI/TRUS fusion biopsy. (**A**,**B**) Peripheral zone target biopsy: (**A**) trans-rectal ultrasound showing the location of the two lesions (orange and blue dots); (**B**) same lesions depicted in a T2-w MR (orange and blue dots). (**C**–**F**) anterior zone target biopsy: (**C**) trans-rectal ultrasound showing the location of the two lesions (orange and blue dots); (**D**) same lesions depicted in a T2-w MR (orange and blue dots); (**E**) fusion image overlapping T2-w MR image on top of transrectal ultrasound (lesions represented as orange and blue dots); (**F**) ADC map of the corresponding lesions.

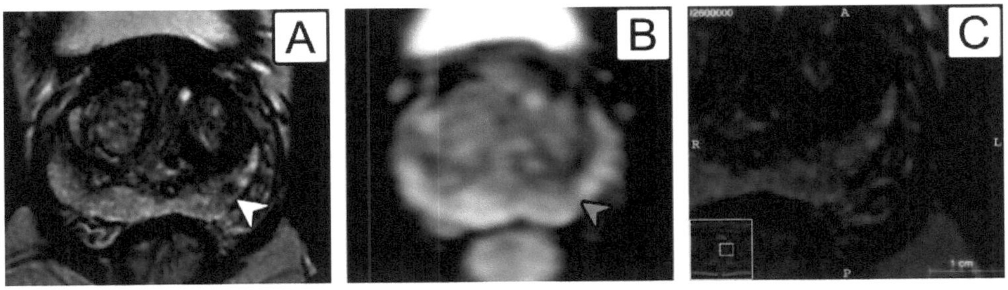

Figure 3. A 64-year-old patient with a PI-RADS 3 lesion in the left mid-gland peripheral zone. (**A**) Lesion on T2-w sequence depicted as a low-signal 5-mm nodule (white arrowhead); (**B**) same lesion highlighted on ADC map (grey arrowhead); (**C**) manual segmentation on ITK-SNAP (red label). Target biopsy revealed fibrosis with focal atrophy without evidence of prostate cancer.

2.5. Reproducible Literature Models Search and Assessment

We searched papers in the literature applying mpMRI radiomics as a tool to identify csPCa among PI-RADS 3 lesions. The following inclusion criteria were used: (1) PI-RADS 3 lesions identified according to PI-RADS v2.1 guidelines; (2) targeted biopsy as ground truth; (3) usage of IBSI-compliant tools for radiomic features computation; (4) adequate description of the methodological details (resampling grid, parameters in radiomic feature computation, selected radiomic features list, and model hyperparameters). Selected works' details are reported in Table 3.

Table 3. Selected models' details.

Reference	Hectors 2021 [16]	Jin 2022 [19]
Number of subjects	240	103
Scanner	3T (GE Signa, Siemens Skyra)	3T (Siemens Skyra)
Endorectal coil	No	No
Radiomics MR sequences	T2	T2, ADC, DWI (1500 mm/s^2)
ROIs	3D (1 operator)	3D (2 operators) on T2 (ADC/DWI registered to T2)
Radiomics platform	Pyradiomics	FeAture Explorer (Pyradiomics)
Intensity normalization	[$\mu - 3\sigma$:$\mu + 3\sigma$] inside the VOI	$(x - \mu)/\sigma$
Resampling	$0.5 \times 0.5 \times 0.5$ mm^3	$1 \times 1 \times 1$ mm^3
Quantization	64 bins	Not specified
Model assessment	Cross-validation + independent test set	Independent test set
Selected radiomic feature details	Yes (20 features)	Yes (4 features)
Clinical parameters in the model	No	Yes (PSA, age)
Model	Random forest with SMOTE	Logistic regression
Radiomics model performances (test set)	AUC 0.76 Sensitivity 75.0% Specificity 79.6%	AUC 0.88 Sensitivity 83% Specificity 65%

We extracted radiomic features from our 80-patient dataset using the work-specific processing and parameters for each work. We assessed the correlation between selected features and biopsy results through a univariate Mann–Whitney test applied to the entire patient sample. Then, pending the trained model availability, we retrained a model with the work-specific attributes and the work-specific input features on our 80-patient dataset, employing 100 repetitions of 5-fold stratified cross-validation and providing results in terms of sensitivity and specificity on the 500 validation sets. The following details are provided.

2.5.1. T2-Based Hectors et al. Model

T2 images were normalized to range between mean $\pm$ 3σ (standard deviation) of the intensity in the volume of interest (VOI), resampled on a $0.5 \times 0.5 \times 0.5$ mm^3 voxel grid, and discretized to 64 bins. The selected 20 radiomic features were used as input in a scikit-learn (https://scikit-learn.org/stable/ (accessed on 17 September 2022)) Random Forest Classifier (maximum depth = 16; maximum number of features = none; minimum number of samples per leaf = 2; minimum number of samples required to split = 2; maximum number of leaf nodes = 16). A SMOTE oversampling of the minority class was adopted.

2.5.2. T2 and DWI-Based Jin et al. Model

T2 and DWI image intensities were standardized; images were then resampled on a $1 \times 1 \times 1$ mm^3 voxel grid. Since the paper did not specify image discretization details, we used Pyradiomics default. The 4 selected radiomic features, along with patient age and PSA, were normalized using Z normalization and given input to a scikit-learn Logistic Regression classifier.

2.6. Proposal of a New Model to Be Validated by Other Centers

As clinical parameters, we assessed PSA, PSA density, age, and mean ADC value within a 2D ROI. Regarding radiomic features, we normalized T2 and ADC images by dividing voxel intensities by the average intensity computed within the corresponding normalization ROI. T2-weighted and ADC volumes were respectively resampled on a $0.4 \times 0.4 \times 3.0$ mm^3 and a $0.8 \times 0.8 \times 3.0$ mm^3 voxel grid through b-spline interpolation. In total, 958 radiomic features per patient were computed with Pyradiomics on original volumes (32 bin quantization) and HHH, LLL, HHL, and LLH coif1 wavelet decompositions (8 bin quantization for T2 and 16 bin quantization for ADC). Clinical and radiomic features more robustly related to GS were selected randomly dividing the 80 patients into 5 groups 100 times (maintaining the csPCa balance). In each of the 500 feature selection trials (4 groups at a time, 64 patients), the Mann–Whitney test assessed the univariate association between clinical/radiomic features and biopsy results. At the same time, we investigated the correlation between features using Spearman rank. The feature with the smallest univariate p-value was firstly selected. Then, features with increasing p values (if $\leq$0.01) were added only if characterized by an absolute value of the Spearman rank correlation <0.5 vs. already selected features. The final selected features pool contains features picked most times out of the 500 trials.

Univariate and multivariate models' definitions and assessments were performed through 100 repetitions of a 5-fold stratified cross-validation scheme. Univariate models were defined by selecting thresholds maximizing the Youden index on training sets (4 groups, 64 patients) and assessed in terms of sensitivity and specificity on validation sets (1 group, 16 patients). The mean and standard deviation of sensitivity and specificity over the 500 validation trials were finally reported for each selected feature. For multivariate analysis, the following six classification models were considered: linear discriminant, linear, quadratic, and cubic support vector machine (SVM), classification tree, and K-nearest neighbours (KNN). All the possible feature combinations from the selected feature pool were assessed as classification model inputs. Models and optimal thresholds were identified on training sets and evaluated in terms of sensitivity and specificity on the corresponding 500 validation sets. Finally, a model to be shared for external validation was trained on the entire dataset. All the analysis was implemented in scikit-learn.

3. Results

Clinical-pathological results are described in Table 1. The detection rate for csPCa (Gleason score $\geq 3 + 4$) at targeted and systematic biopsies in the case of PI-RADS 3, 4, and 5 was 32, 46, and 67%, respectively.

3.1. Assessment of Literature Features/Models

In Table 4, we reported the univariate association between radiomic features contained in Hectors' [16] and Jin's [19] models and biopsy results in our 80-patient dataset.

Table 4. Univariate association between radiomic features contained in Hectors's [16] and Jin's [19] models and biopsy results in our 80-patient dataset; features with p-value ≤ 0.05 are in bold.

Hector's Features	p-Value
T2-original_shape_Elongation	0.13
T2-original_shape_Flatness	0.14
T2-original_firstorder_10Percentile	0.94
T2-original_firstorder_InterquartileRange	0.40
T2-original_firstorder_Mean	0.43
T2-original_firstorder_Median	0.51
T2-original_firstorder_RootMeanSquared	0.38
T2-original_glcm_Autocorrelation	**0.01**
T2-original_glcm_DifferenceEntropy	0.06
T2-original_glcm_InverseVariance	**0.02**
T2-original_glcm_JointAverage	**0.01**
T2-original_glcm_JointEnergy	**0.04**
T2-original_gldm_LargeDependenceLowGrayLevelEmphasis	0.10
T2-original_glrlm_LongRunEmphasis	**0.05**
T2-original_glrlm_LongRunHighGrayLevelEmphasis	**0.01**
T2-original_glszm_GrayLevelVariance	0.12
T2-original_glszm_SizeZoneNonUniformity	**0.03**
T2-original_glszm_SmallAreaEmphasis	**0.01**
T2-original_ngtdm_Complexity	0.27
T2-original-ngtdm_Strength	**0.05**
Jin's Features	**p-Value**
T2-wavelet-HHL_glcm_ClusterTendency	**0.005**
DWI-original_glcm_ldmn	0.74
DWI-wavelet-LLL_glrlm_LongRunLowGrayLevelEmphasis	0.11
DWI-wavelet-LLL glszm_SizeZoneNonUniformityNormalized	0.75

Regarding the performance of the re-implemented multivariate models relying on these features, Hector's random forest model obtained a sensitivity of 40% ± 21% and a specificity of 71% ± 15%. Jin's logistic regression model, which combined radiomic features, age, and PSA, obtained a sensitivity of 36% ± 20% and a specificity of 89% ± 10%.

3.2. Proposed Model

In the 500 feature selection trials, features more often selected and, therefore, more robustly correlated with biopsy were the following: (a) PSA Density (selection rate 100%); (b) a radiomic texture feature computed on the LLL wavelet band of T2-weighted images (T2-wavelet-LLL_glcm_InverseVariance, selection rate 87%); (c) a radiomic texture feature computed on the LLL wavelet band of ADC maps (ADC-wavelet-LLL_glszm_SizeZoneNonUniformity, selection rate 83%).The results of the univariate models' assessment of the 500 validation trials are shown in Table 5. The correlation with histology was as follows: PSA density 66% ± 21% sensitivity and 71% ± 13% specificity; RF-T2 74% ± 21% sensitivity and 55% ± 15% specificity; RF-ADC 44% ± 19% sensitivity and 83% ± 13% specificity. In Table 5, the results obtained by the best multivariate model are also shown. The best multivariate model was a linear discriminant with the three features in input, which obtained a sensitivity of 80% ± 18% and a specificity of 76% ± 13% on the 500 test trials.

Table 5. Selected features and performance of univariate and best multivariate models.

	Selection Rate	Sensitivity	Specificity
PSA Density	100%	66% ± 21%	71% ± 13%
T2-wavelet-LLL_glcm_InverseVariance	87%	74% ± 21%	55% ± 15%
ADC-wavelet-LLL_glszm_SizeZoneNonUniformity	83%	44% ± 19%	83% ± 13%
Trivariate linear discriminant model	-	80% ± 18%	76% ± 13%

4. Discussion

Two works on mpMRI radiomics in prostate cancer recently showed that single-center models' performance drops when models are applied to other center data [22,23]. This may be due to the too-small size of the training sample and to differences among centers in MR scanners, acquisition parameters, histological analysis, and segmentation. Protocol standardization, data, and model sharing will hopefully improve models' reproducibility in the near future. Meanwhile, a step forward toward model generalizability assessment can be made as follows: (1) trying to test radiomics models proposed by others on an external dataset; (2) properly detailing radiomics works so that other groups can assess them on their own data. Unfortunately, to date, few groups in the literature have tested radiomic models developed by other centers. This is often due to the partial lack of details in radiomic papers, which prevents model re-implementation.

In this work, first, we tried to apply reproducible and standard-compliant literature research papers on mpMRI radiomics for PI-RADS 3 csPCa identification on our 80-patient dataset. We reviewed and summarized parameters, methodological choices, and results to simplify further validation by other groups. Then, we proposed a fully detailed and easily implementable new model for assessment on an external dataset. The following two works in literature satisfied our inclusion criteria: one from Hectors et al. [16], who proposed a T2-based model, and one from Jin et al. [19], who proposed a model relying on T2, DWI, age, and PSA. In total, 9 of the 20 radiomic features identified by Hectors et al. resulted significantly correlated to biopsy in our dataset (p-value ranging from 0.01 to 0.05), and 1 of the 4 radiomic features identified by Jin et al. resulted very significantly related to biopsy in our dataset (p-value 0.005). These features are all computed on T2 images, where peripheral and transitional zone lesion contours are easier to delineate and, therefore, likely less user-dependent.

In developing our radiomic model, we performed methodological choices that differed from the two groups. Mainly, we normalized intensities through a peripheral zone normalization ROI (as suggested by Bonekamp et al., 2018 [28]) and applied an FBN quantization with 32 bins on original images, 16 bins on ADC wavelet sub-bands, and 8 bins on T2 wavelet sub-bands. Other normalization/quantization schemes provided worse results and were not shown. The two radiomic features we found most robustly related to biopsy are both computed on the LLL wavelet sub-band, i.e., on a spatially smoothed version of T2 and ADC intensities inside the lesions.

The first feature, T2-wavelet-LLL_glcm_InverseVariance, reflects texture regularity. It was lower than 0.47 on csPCa, thus indicating that clinically significant tumors are characterized by a larger texture irregularity in the low-frequency sub-band of T2 images. This feature alone has good sensitivity (74%) but low specificity (55%). The second feature, ADC-wavelet-LLL_glszm_SizeZoneNonUniformity, measures the variability in the volumes of lesion zones (groups of connected voxels with similar intensity). It was larger than 17 on csPCa, thus indicating their more extensive zone size heterogeneity. This feature alone has a reasonable specificity (83%) but a low sensitivity (44%). It is worth noticing that the normalized version of this feature, computed on DWI, correlated to biopsy in the work of Jin. The lack of significance of Jin's DWI feature on our dataset may be due to differences in the DWI acquisition protocol as follows: we used a b-value of 2000 mm/s^2, while Jin used a b-value of 1500 mm/s^2. We can therefore observe the following: (1) there is a coherence between our result and Jin's; therefore, a greater zone size heterogeneity at the microstructural level is more likely related to malignancy; (2) the computation of this feature on ADC maps may be more robust and repeatable, being less dependent on DWI acquisition b-value.

Similarly to Jin et al., we then developed a multivariate model relying on radiomic and clinical features. However, we did not select clinical and radiomic features independently but included both within a single pool, to which a feature selection strategy was applied. Among clinical features, we selected PSA density, as alone might help tumor discrimination [29] (sensitivity of 66%, specificity of 71% in our dataset). A tri-variate model built on PSA density and the two readily available T2 and ADC radiomic features appears to discriminate csPCa with good confidence (sensitivity of 80%, specificity of 76%). We provided all the methodological details and are available to share trained models and optimized thresholds for external validation.

The model we are proposing is based on bi-parametric MRI (T2 and ADC sequences only, which are routinely acquired). It does not require time-consuming sequences, such as DCE images, which also expose patients to contrast medium-related possible side effects in an effort to build the simplest possible model able to identify csPCa, with the added benefit of reducing segmentation times and guaranteeing better standardization, thereby reducing the possible impact introduced by different DCE acquisition protocols and segmentation methods. Additionally, our model is based only on the following three features: the PSA density (routinely obtained in the standard workup of these patients) and the two radiomic features obtained in two standard mpMRI studies. We are aware that, in machine learning, wrapped and embedded feature selection methods that optimally combine a broader number of features within model optimization or even deep learning models, as seen in Bertelli et al. [30], are often used. However, we preferred to follow a different approach to try to obtain an explainable radiomic model, i.e., one able to explain lesion characteristics related to malignancy.

We think this approach has relevant implications in driving the adoption of radiomics in the clinical management of PI-RADS 3 lesions. From a radiological standpoint, it might complement the radiologist's evaluation, increasing the overall diagnostic accuracy; on the other hand, from a clinical perspective, it might allow us to rule out unnecessary biopsies, avoiding the risk of procedure-related possible complications in selected patients.

This study has several limitations, mainly the small number of patients and the lack of an independent testing dataset. However, we tried to provide results as robustly as possible by performing both feature selection and model assessment in multiple subsamples. Furthermore, it is necessary to recognize that the pathological standard of reference should be the radical prostatectomy sample, not the histological result of the biopsy. In fact, our recent experience has shown that the combination of target and systematic biopsies fails to detect about 15% of the foci of csPCa at definitive pathology. However, only 4% turned out to be the index lesion (data not yet published). It could also be argued that the method used at our Institution for targeted biopsies is a rigid fusion, while there are elastic fusion technologies that can allow more accurate targeting. However, in a recent systematic review and meta-analysis, no significant difference in the detection of csPCa was identified when comparing rigid and elastic registration for MRI-TRUS fusion-guided biopsy [31].

Moreover, the high PI-RADS 3 lesion prevalence in the peripheral zone (82.5%) did not allow an investigation of any possible zone-related difference, and the overall sample size did not allow us to evaluate sector-related differences. We think there is a need for future research to assess not only regional differences between the transitional and peripheral zones but also different sectors' related variability. Not clinically significant prostate cancers (Gleason score 3 + 3) were included in the negative group, as data in this last category were not conspicuous. However, this choice does not imply a particularly significant clinical limitation. MRI follow-up, with or without biopsy mapping, is usually performed for PI-RADS 3 lesions. Lastly, since the dataset was quite imbalanced (32.5% of tumors), we decided to optimize thresholds instead of using SMOTE since optimal thresholds provided better results.

5. Conclusions

Standard-compliant works with robust and detailed methodologies achieve comparable radiomic feature sets. Therefore, efforts to facilitate external validation of csPCa identification models with independent datasets are needed to help radiomics gain an effective role in the clinical workflow. In contrast, complex imaging models and protocols do not seem to be required. We showed indeed that PSA density, combined with two radiomic features computed on two routinely performed sequences (T2 and ADC), may potentially discriminate clinically significant prostate cancers (Gleason score $\geq 3 + 4$).

Author Contributions: Conceptualization, A.C., E.D.B. and P.A.B.; methodology, A.C., E.D.B. and P.A.B.; software, E.D.B.; validation, E.D.B.; formal analysis, E.D.B.; investigation, A.C., E.D.B. and P.N.F.; resources, A.C., P.A.B. and P.N.F.; data curation, A.C., E.D.B., P.A.B., P.N.F., D.N., R.S. and G.P.; writing—original draft preparation, A.C., E.D.B., P.A.B. and D.N.; writing—review and editing, A.C., E.D.B., P.A.B., P.N.F., D.I., G.P., M.R., M.O., L.F.D.P. and S.S.; visualization, A.C., E.D.B., P.A.B., P.N.F., D.N., R.S., D.I., M.R. and M.O.; supervision, L.F.D.P. and S.S.; project administration, S.S. All authors have read and agreed to the published version of the manuscript.

Funding: This research received no external funding.

Institutional Review Board Statement: The study was conducted in accordance with the Declaration of Helsinki and approved by the local Institutional Review Board of ASST Papa Giovanni XXIII Bergamo (protocol code 'mpMR e Sorveglianza Attiva', 7 June 2018).

Informed Consent Statement: Informed consent was obtained from all subjects involved in the study.

Data Availability Statement: The data presented in this study are available on request from the corresponding author.

Conflicts of Interest: The authors declare no conflict of interest.

References

1. Torre, L.A.; Bray, F.; Siegel, R.L.; Ferlay, J.; Lortet-Tieulent, J.; Jemal, A. Global cancer statistics, 2012. *CA Cancer J. Clin.* **2015**, *65*, 87–108. [CrossRef] [PubMed]
2. Delongchamps, N.B.; Rouanne, M.; Flam, T.; Beuvon, F.; Liberatore, M.; Zerbib, M.; Cornud, F. Multiparametric magnetic resonance imaging for the detection and localization of prostate cancer: Combination of T2-weighted, dynamic contrast-enhanced and diffusion-weighted imaging: Increased prostate cancer detection with multiparametric MRI. *BJU Int.* **2011**, *107*, 1411–1418. [CrossRef] [PubMed]
3. Turkbey, B.; Rosenkrantz, A.B.; Haider, M.A.; Padhani, A.R.; Villeirs, G.; Macura, K.J.; Tempany, C.M.; Choyke, P.L.; Cornud, F.; Margolis, D.J.; et al. Prostate Imaging Reporting and Data System Version 2.1: 2019 Update of Prostate Imaging Reporting and Data System Version 2. *Eur. Urol.* **2019**, *76*, 340–351. [CrossRef]
4. Tamada, T.; Sone, T.; Jo, Y.; Toshimitsu, S.; Yamashita, T.; Yamamoto, A.; Tanimoto, D.; Ito, K. Apparent diffusion coefficient values in peripheral and transition zones of the prostate: Comparison between normal and malignant prostatic tissues and correlation with histologic grade. *J. Magn. Reson. Imaging* **2008**, *28*, 720–726. [CrossRef] [PubMed]
5. Nagarajan, R.; Margolis, D.; Raman, S.; Sheng, K.; King, C.; Reiter, R.; Thomas, M.A. Correlation of Gleason Scores with Diffusion-Weighted Imaging Findings of Prostate Cancer. *Adv. Urol.* **2012**, *2012*, 374805. [CrossRef]
6. Hambrock, T.; Somford, D.M.; Huisman, H.J.; van Oort, I.M.; Witjes, J.A.; Hulsbergen-van de Kaa, C.A.; Scheenen, T.; Barentsz, J.O. Relationship between Apparent Diffusion Coefficients at 3.0-T MR Imaging and Gleason Grade in Peripheral Zone Prostate Cancer. *Radiology* **2011**, *259*, 453–461. [CrossRef]
7. Kitajima, K.; Takahashi, S.; Ueno, Y.; Miyake, H.; Fujisawa, M.; Kawakami, F.; Sugimura, K. Do apparent diffusion coefficient (ADC) values obtained using high b-values with a 3-T MRI correlate better than a transrectal ultrasound (TRUS)-guided biopsy with true Gleason scores obtained from radical prostatectomy specimens for patients with prostate cancer? *Eur. J. Radiol.* **2013**, *82*, 1219–1226. [CrossRef]

8. Kasivisvanathan, V.; Rannikko, A.S.; Borghi, M.; Panebianco, V.; Mynderse, L.A.; Vaarala, M.H.; Briganti, A.; Budäus, L.; Hellawell, G.; Hindley, R.G.; et al. MRI-Targeted or Standard Biopsy for Prostate-Cancer Diagnosis. *N. Engl. J. Med.* **2018**, *378*, 1767–1777. [CrossRef]
9. Schoots, I.G. MRI in early prostate cancer detection: How to manage indeterminate or equivocal PI-RADS 3 lesions? *Transl. Androl. Urol.* **2018**, *7*, 70–82. [CrossRef]
10. Padhani, A.R.; Barentsz, J.; Villeirs, G.; Rosenkrantz, A.B.; Margolis, D.J.; Turkbey, B.; Thoeny, H.C.; Cornud, F.; Haider, M.A.; Macura, K.J.; et al. PI-RADS Steering Committee: The PI-RADS Multiparametric MRI and MRI-directed Biopsy Pathway. *Radiology* **2019**, *292*, 464–474. [CrossRef]
11. Epstein, J.I.; Egevad, L.; Amin, M.B.; Delahunt, B.; Srigley, J.R.; Humphrey, P.A.; Grading Committee. The 2014 International Society of Urological Pathology (ISUP) Consensus Conference on Gleason Grading of Prostatic Carcinoma: Definition of Grading Patterns and Proposal for a New Grading System. *Am. J. Surg. Pathol.* **2016**, *40*, 244–252. [CrossRef]
12. Greer, M.D.; Brown, A.M.; Shih, J.H.; Summers, R.M.; Marko, J.; Law, Y.M.; Sankineni, S.; George, A.K.; Merino, M.J.; Pinto, P.A.; et al. Accuracy and agreement of PIRADSv2 for prostate cancer mpMRI: A multireader study: PIRADSv2 for Prostate Tumor Detection. *J. Magn. Reson. Imaging* **2017**, *45*, 579–585. [CrossRef]
13. Hansen, N.L.; Kesch, C.; Barrett, T.; Koo, B.; Radtke, J.P.; Bonekamp, D.; Schlemmer, H.-P.; Warren, A.Y.; Wieczorek, K.; Hohenfellner, M.; et al. Multicentre evaluation of targeted and systematic biopsies using magnetic resonance and ultrasound image-fusion guided transperineal prostate biopsy in patients with a previous negative biopsy. *BJU Int.* **2017**, *120*, 631–638. [CrossRef] [PubMed]
14. Giambelluca, D.; Cannella, R.; Vernuccio, F.; Comelli, A.; Pavone, A.; Salvaggio, L.; Galia, M.; Midiri, M.; Lagalla, R.; Salvaggio, G. PI-RADS 3 Lesions: Role of Prostate MRI Texture Analysis in the Identification of Prostate Cancer. *Curr. Probl. Diagn. Radiol.* **2021**, *50*, 175–185. [CrossRef] [PubMed]
15. Hou, Y.; Bao, M.-L.; Wu, C.-J.; Zhang, J.; Zhang, Y.-D.; Shi, H.-B. A radiomics machine learning-based redefining score robustly identifies clinically significant prostate cancer in equivocal PI-RADS score 3 lesions. *Abdom. Radiol.* **2020**, *45*, 4223–4234. [CrossRef] [PubMed]
16. Hectors, S.J.; Chen, C.; Chen, J.; Wang, J.; Gordon, S.; Yu, M.; Al Hussein Al Awamlh, B.; Sabuncu, M.R.; Margolis, D.J.A.; Hu, J.C. Magnetic Resonance Imaging Radiomics-Based Machine Learning Prediction of Clinically Significant Prostate Cancer in Equivocal PI-RADS 3 Lesions. *J. Magn. Reson. Imaging* **2021**, *54*, 1466–1473. [CrossRef]
17. Brancato, V.; Aiello, M.; Basso, L.; Monti, S.; Palumbo, L.; Di Costanzo, G.; Salvatore, M.; Ragozzino, A.; Cavaliere, C. Evaluation of a multiparametric MRI radiomic-based approach for stratification of equivocal PI-RADS 3 and upgraded PI-RADS 4 prostatic lesions. *Sci. Rep.* **2021**, *11*, 643. [CrossRef]
18. Lim, C.S.; Abreu-Gomez, J.; Thornhill, R.; James, N.; Al Kindi, A.; Lim, A.S.; Schieda, N. Utility of machine learning of apparent diffusion coefficient (ADC) and T2-weighted (T2W) radiomic features in PI-RADS version 2.1 category 3 lesions to predict prostate cancer diagnosis. *Abdom. Radiol.* **2021**, *46*, 5647–5658. [CrossRef]
19. Jin, P.; Yang, L.; Qiao, X.; Hu, C.; Hu, C.; Wang, X.; Bao, J. Utility of Clinical-Radiomic Model to Identify Clinically Significant Prostate Cancer in Biparametric MRI PI-RADS V2.1 Category 3 Lesions. *Front. Oncol.* **2022**, *12*, 840786. [CrossRef]
20. Ferro, M.; de Cobelli, O.; Musi, G.; Del Giudice, F.; Carrieri, G.; Busetto, G.M.; Falagario, U.G.; Sciarra, A.; Maggi, M.; Crocetto, F.; et al. Radiomics in prostate cancer: An up-to-date review. *Adv. Urol.* **2022**, *14*, 17562872221109020. [CrossRef]
21. Liu, X.; Elbanan, M.G.; Luna, A.; Haider, M.A.; Smith, A.D.; Sabottke, C.F.; Spieler, B.M.; Turkbey, B.; Fuentes, D.; Moawad, A.; et al. Radiomics in Abdominopelvic Solid-Organ Oncologic Imaging: Current Status. *AJR Am. J. Roentgenol.* **2022**. *preprint*. [CrossRef] [PubMed]
22. Castillo, T.J.M.; Starmans, M.P.A.; Arif, M.; Niessen, W.J.; Klein, S.; Bangma, C.H.; Schoots, I.G.; Veenland, J.F. A Multi-Center, Multi-Vendor Study to Evaluate the Generalizability of a Radiomics Model for Classifying Prostate cancer: High Grade vs. Low Grade. *Diagnostics* **2021**, *11*, 369. [CrossRef] [PubMed]
23. Bleker, J.; Yakar, D.; van Noort, B.; Rouw, D.; de Jong, I.J.; Dierckx, R.A.J.O.; Kwee, T.C.; Huisman, H. Single-center versus multi-center biparametric MRI radiomics approach for clinically significant peripheral zone prostate cancer. *Insights Imaging* **2021**, *12*, 150. [CrossRef] [PubMed]
24. Zwanenburg, A.; Vallières, M.; Abdalah, M.A.; Aerts, H.J.W.L.; Andrearczyk, V.; Apte, A.; Ashrafinia, S.; Bakas, S.; Beukinga, R.J.; Boellaard, R.; et al. The Image Biomarker Standardization Initiative: Standardized Quantitative Radiomics for High-Throughput Image-based Phenotyping. *Radiology* **2020**, *295*, 328–338. [CrossRef]
25. Hansen, N.; Patruno, G.; Wadhwa, K.; Gaziev, G.; Miano, R.; Barrett, T.; Gnanapragasam, V.; Doble, A.; Warren, A.; Bratt, O.; et al. Magnetic Resonance and Ultrasound Image Fusion Supported Transperineal Prostate Biopsy Using the Ginsburg Protocol: Technique, Learning Points, and Biopsy Results. *Eur. Urol.* **2016**, *70*, 332–340. [CrossRef]
26. Epstein, J.I.; Allsbrook, W.C.; Amin, M.B.; Egevad, L.L.; ISUP Grading Committee. The 2005 International Society of Urological Pathology (ISUP) Consensus Conference on Gleason Grading of Prostatic Carcinoma. *Am. J. Surg. Pathol.* **2005**, *29*, 1228–1242. [CrossRef] [PubMed]
27. Yushkevich, P.A.; Piven, J.; Hazlett, H.C.; Smith, R.G.; Ho, S.; Gee, J.C.; Gerig, G. User-guided 3D active contour segmentation of anatomical structures: Significantly improved efficiency and reliability. *NeuroImage* **2006**, *31*, 1116–1128. [CrossRef]

28. Bonekamp, D.; Kohl, S.; Wiesenfarth, M.; Schelb, P.; Radtke, J.P.; Götz, M.; Kickingereder, P.; Yaqubi, K.; Hitthaler, B.; Gählert, N.; et al. Radiomic Machine Learning for Characterization of Prostate Lesions with MRI: Comparison to ADC Values. *Radiology* **2018**, *289*, 128–137. [CrossRef]
29. Roscigno, M.; Stabile, A.; Lughezzani, G.; Pepe, P.; Galosi, A.B.; Naselli, A.; Naspro, R.; Nicolai, M.; La Croce, G.; Aljoulani, M.; et al. The Use of Multiparametric Magnetic Resonance Imaging for Follow-up of Patients Included in Active Surveillance Protocol. Can PSA Density Discriminate Patients at Different Risk of Reclassification? *Clin. Genitourin. Cancer* **2020**, *18*, e698–e704. [CrossRef]
30. Bertelli, E.; Mercatelli, L.; Marzi, C.; Pachetti, E.; Baccini, M.; Barucci, A.; Colantonio, S.; Gherardini, L.; Lattavo, L.; Pascali, M.A.; et al. Machine and Deep Learning Prediction of Prostate Cancer Aggressiveness Using Multiparametric MRI. *Front. Oncol.* **2021**, *11*, 802964. [CrossRef]
31. Venderink, W.; de Rooij, M.; Sedelaar, J.P.M.; Huisman, H.J.; Fütterer, J.J. Elastic Versus Rigid Image Registration in Magnetic Resonance Imaging-Transrectal Ultrasound Fusion Prostate Biopsy: A Systematic Review and Meta-Analysis. *Eur. Urol. Focus* **2018**, *4*, 219–227. [CrossRef] [PubMed]

Journal of
Clinical Medicine

MDPI

Article

Predictors of Clinically Significant Prostate Cancer in Patients with PIRADS Categories 3–5 Undergoing Magnetic Resonance Imaging-Ultrasound Fusion Biopsy of the Prostate

Stanisław Szempliński [1,2], Hubert Kamecki [1,*], Małgorzata Dębowska [3,4], Bartłomiej Zagożdżon [1], Mateusz Mokrzyś [5], Marek Zawadzki [5], Roman Sosnowski [6], Andrzej Tokarczyk [1], Sławomir Poletajew [1], Piotr Kryst [1] and Łukasz Nyk [1]

1 Second Department of Urology, Centre of Postgraduate Medical Education, 01-809 Warsaw, Poland
2 Medyczne Centrum Diagnostyczne Voxel, 00-671 Warsaw, Poland
3 Nałęcz Institute of Biocybernetics and Biomedical Engineering, Polish Academy of Sciences, 02-109 Warsaw, Poland
4 Department of Computational Oncology, Maria Skłodowska-Curie National Research Institute of Oncology, 02-781 Warsaw, Poland
5 Department of Urology, St. Anna Hospital, 05-500 Piaseczno, Poland
6 Department of Urogenital Cancer, Maria Skłodowska-Curie National Research Institute of Oncology, 02-781 Warsaw, Poland
* Correspondence: hubert.kamecki@ecz-otwock.pl

Abstract: Prostate biopsy is recommended in cases of positive magnetic resonance imaging (MRI), defined as Prostate Imaging Reporting and Data System (PIRADS) category ≥ 3. However, most men with positive MRIs will not be diagnosed with clinically significant prostate cancer (csPC). Our goal was to evaluate pre-biopsy characteristics that influence the probability of a csPC diagnosis in these patients. We retrospectively analyzed 740 consecutive men with a positive MRI and no prior PC diagnosis who underwent MRI-ultrasound fusion biopsies of the prostate in three centers. csPC detection rates (CDRs) for each PIRADS category were calculated. Patient, disease, and lesion characteristics were studied for interdependencies with the csPC diagnosis. The CDR in patients with PIRADS categories 3, 4, and 5 was 10.5%, 30.7%, and 54.6%, respectively. On both uni- and multivariable regression models, older age, being biopsy-naïve, prostate specific antigen ≥ 10 ng/mL, smaller prostate volume, PIRADS > 3, a larger maximum lesion size, a lesion in the peripheral zone, and a positive digital rectal examination were associated with csPC. In this large, multicenter study, we provide new data regarding CDRs in particular PIRADS categories. In addition, we present several strong predictors that further alter the risk of csPC in MRI-positive patients. Our results could help in refining individual risk assessment, especially in PIRADS 3 patients, in whom the risk of csPC is substantially low.

Keywords: detection rate; multiparametric magnetic resonance imaging; positive predictive value; prostate imaging reporting and data system version 2; prostate cancer; targeted biopsy

1. Introduction

Prostate cancer (PC) is the second most commonly diagnosed male malignancy [1], with mortality reaching approximately 375,000 annual deaths worldwide [2]. The likelihood of unfavorable outcomes strongly depends on individual cancer pathology, which has led to the development of the concept of clinically significant PC (csPC), which, contrary to low-risk PC, which is eligible for active surveillance, should be managed with active treatment. Many strategies have been aimed at tailoring the overall PC diagnosis yield to csPC cases only, with current data showing that the rates of men diagnosed with low-risk PC are on a downtrend [3]. The core initial risk stratification tool is magnetic resonance imaging (MRI) of the prostate and assessment with the Prostate Imaging Reporting and

Data System (PIRADS) [4], with MRI-guided needle biopsies of the prostate allowing for the most accurate assessment of tumor pathology [5]. As recommended by the European Association of Urology, a prostate biopsy should be performed in cases of positive MRI, defined as PIRADS category 3 or higher [6].

However, contemporary data shows that most patients with a positive MRI who undergo prostate biopsy will not be diagnosed with csPC [7]. Thus, a positive MRI alone cannot be considered a strong predictor of a csPC diagnosis, and other risk factors should be pursued. In order to provide data that could help in refining individual risk assessment, the aim of this study was to retrospectively analyze a large cohort of MRI-positive patients who underwent MRI-ultrasound fusion biopsy of the prostate in order to provide csPC detection rates (cancer detection rates, CDR) for PIRADS categories 3, 4, and 5, as well as to study possible associations between specific patient or lesion characteristics and an increase in the risk of csPC.

2. Materials and Methods

We retrospectively analyzed consecutive patients without a prior history of PC who underwent MRI-ultrasound fusion biopsies of the prostate at three centers, including one university hospital, between March 2018 and October 2021. Data were collected from medical patient records and included: age, previous medical history, pre-biopsy prostate-specific antigen (PSA) level, MRI report, biopsy procedure report, and pathology report. The study included patients with PIRADS category 3 or higher. Patients with incomplete data were excluded from the study.

2.1. MRI-Ultrasound Fusion Biopsy

An MRI was performed either at our institutions or externally, with external studies having been reviewed by an institutional radiologist in case of ambiguities. PIRADS version 2.0 or 2.1 was used in all cases. All biopsies were performed with the KOELIS Trinity MRI/US OBT Fusion® system, using either a transperineal or transrectal approach. Two experienced urologists, without the assistance of another physician, performed all the procedures at the three participating centers. A digital rectal examination (DRE) was carried out and recorded just before the procedure. The selection of the biopsy approach (transperineal or transrectal) was primarily indicated by individual urologist expertise, with the transperineal approach being preferred in order to reduce the risk of infectious complications. Transperineal biopsies were performed with the aid of the KOELIS Full Grid™ device. Every biopsy included cores targeted at all the PIRADS ≥ 3 lesions identified in the MRI report. The number of targeted cores was never less than 3 per lesion, as defined by the policy the urologists adhered to. A greater number of targeted cores might have been taken if deemed necessary by the urologist. Occasionally, the biopsy may have also included additional cores targeted at lesions not identified in the report but considered suspicious by the performing urologist or the reviewing radiologist. In all biopsy-naïve patients, systematic cores were included. In patients with a previous negative biopsy, the addition of systematic cores was at the discretion of the urologist. Systematic cores, if included, did not cover the regions subject to targeted biopsy. The number of systematic cores was at the discretion of the urologist, being dependent predominantly on the lesion location and prostate volume. All the specimens were assessed by institutional pathologists. All the pathologists were specialists in urogenital cancer and adhered to the International Society of Urological Pathology (ISUP) guidelines.

2.2. Definitions

We defined a csPC diagnosis as the presence of grade group ≥ 2 cancer in either targeted or systematic cores. To represent a typical clinical scenario, we defined the highest PIRADS category as the highest category of a lesion as classified by the radiologist in the original MRI report, regardless of the performing urologist's or reviewing institutional radiologist's second opinion. The maximum lesion size was the size of the largest lesion in the highest PIRADS category in a patient. The number of cores was the total number of cores taken during the biopsy procedure.

2.3. Outcome Measurements and Statistical Analysis

Categorical and quantitative variables were calculated as numbers with percentages and medians (with interquartile ranges), respectively. The associations between categorical and continuous variables and a dependent variable were investigated using univariable and multivariable logistic regression models. The outcomes of logistic regression models were expressed as odds ratios (OR) with 95% confidence intervals (95% CIs). Results were considered statistically significant at a p-value < 0.05. Statistical analyses were performed using MATLAB R2021a (MathWorks, Natick, MA, USA) and R version 4.0.3 (R Foundation for Statistical Computing, Vienna, Austria).

3. Results

We identified 748 patients who met the inclusion criteria. Eight patients were excluded due to incomplete data. Eventually, 740 men were enrolled into the analyses. Data, including baseline patient and lesion characteristics, biopsy approach, median number of cores, and csPC diagnosis rate, are presented in Table 1.

Table 1. Characteristics of patients

Characteristic	All Patients (n = 740)	Center 1 (n = 298)	Center 2 (n = 122)	Center 3 (n = 320)
Median age, years (IQR)	65 (60, 69)	64 (58, 69)	66 (62, 69)	65 (61, 69)
Biopsy-naïve (%)	416 (56.2)	165 (55.4)	56 (45.9)	195 (60.9)
Median PSA, ng/mL (IQR)	6.9 (4.9, 9.7)	7.0 (5.1, 10.0)	7.5 (5.4, 10.0)	6.2 (4.7–9.1)
Median PV, mL (IQR)	42.7 (33.1, 59.7)	41.0 (32.8, 55.9)	48.9 (37.3, 63.0)	42.4 (33.0, 60.0)
Median max. lesion size, mm (IQR)	13 (10, 17)	13 (10, 16)	14 (10, 18)	13 (9, 16)
PIRADS category (%)				
3	124 (16.8)	63 (21.1)	11 (9.0)	50 (15.6)
4	398 (53.8)	144 (48.3)	66 (54.1)	188 (58.8)
5	218 (29.5)	91 (30.5)	45 (36.9)	82 (25.6)
Lesion in the peripheral zone (%)	485 (69.6) [a]	158 (62.0) [a]	101 (82.8)	226 (70.1)
Positive DRE [b]	131 (18.5) [b]	56 (21.0) [b]	13 (10.7)	62 (19.4)
Biopsy approach, n				
Transperineal	615 (83.1)	182 (61.1)	113 (92.4)	320 (100.0)
Transrectal	125 (16.9)	116 (38.9)	9 (7.6)	0 (0.0)
Median number of cores (IQR)	11 (9, 15)	17 (16, 19)	19 (18, 23)	11 (9, 14)
Diagnosis of csPC (%)	254 (34.3)	114 (38.3)	35 (28.7)	105 (32.8)

IQR, interquartile range; PSA, prostate-specific antigen; PV—prostate volume; PIRADS—prostate imaging reporting and data system; DRE, digital rectal examination; csPC, or clinically significant prostate cancer. Center 1 was university-affiliated. [a] Data lacking for 43 patients, percentages calculated for known data. [b] Data lacking for 31 patients, percentages were calculated using known data.

The CDR in patients with PIRADS categories 3, 4, and 5 was 10.5% (95% CI: 5.1–15.9%), 30.7% (95% CI: 26.1–35.2), and 54.6% (95% CI: 48.0–61.2%), respectively (Figure 1).

The type of biopsy approach (transrectal or transperineal) was not associated with the probability of a csPC diagnosis (CDRs: 37.6 vs. 33.7%, respectively, $p = 0.75$).

Concerning univariable analysis, older age, being biopsy-naïve, having a PSA level $\geq$ 10 ng/mL, a smaller prostate volume, a PIRADS category > 3, a larger maximum lesion size, a lesion located in the peripheral zone (PZ), and a positive digital rectal examination (DRE) were associated with an increased risk of csPC diagnosis (Table 2). All these variables were then included in a multivariable model, demonstrating a significant association with csPC (Table 2) as well.

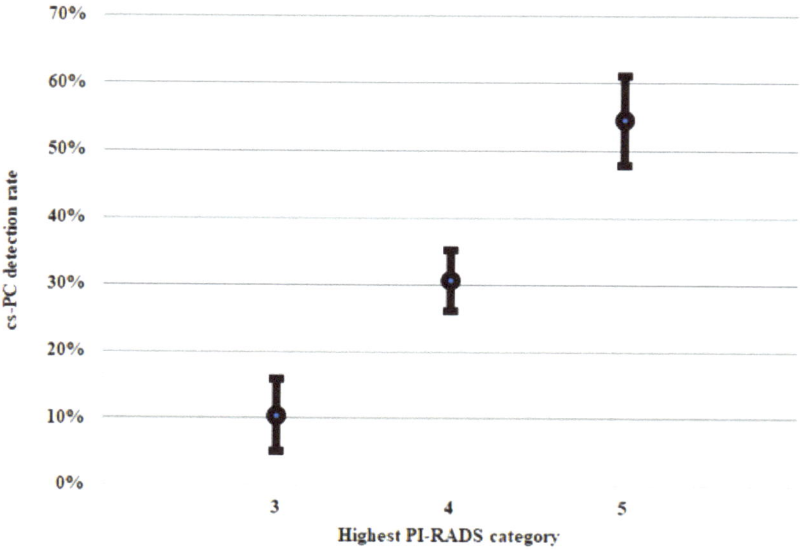

Figure 1. Detection rates of clinically significant prostate cancer (cs-PC) among patients with the highest Prostate Imaging Reporting and Data System (PIRADS) categories 3, 4, and 5. The whiskers represent 95% confidence intervals.

Table 2. Association between clinically significant prostate cancer (csPC) diagnosis and other factors, DRE included.

	UVA vs. csPC OR (95% CI), *p*-Value	MVA vs. csPC OR (95% CI), *p*-Value
Age, years	1.05 (1.03–1.07), <0.001	1.05 (1.03–1.08), <0.001
Biopsy-naïve	1.42 (1.04–1.93), 0.027	1.57 (1.08–2.29), 0.017
PSA > 10 ng/mL	2.57 (1.81–3.65), <0.001	2.36 (1.53–3.64), <0.001
PV, mL	0.98 (0.98–0.99), <0.001	0.98 (0.97–0.98), <0.001
Max. lesion size, mm	1.07 (1.05–1.10), <0.001	1.05 (1.02–1.08), 0.001
PIRADS > 3	5.49 (3.02–9.10), <0.001	3.14 (1.63–6.05), 0.001
Lesion in PZ	2.05 (1.43–2.95), <0.001	1.86 (1.24–2.79), 0.003
Positive DRE	3.14 (2.12–4.63), <0.001	1.74 (1.12–2.70), 0.014

UVA, univariable analysis; MVA, multivariable analysis (logistic regression model, n = 697); OR, odds ratio; CI, confidence interval; PSA, prostate-specific antigen; PIRADS, prostate imaging reporting, and data system; PZ, peripheral zone; DRE, digital rectal examination.

Considering the possibility of observer bias when interpreting the DRE result, we developed another multivariable logistic regression model that did not include DRE; the statistical significance of the associations between the remaining variables and the dependent variable became even stronger (Table 3).

We performed a similar multivariable analysis limited to patients with the highest PIRADS category 3. In both models (DRE included and DRE excluded), only a smaller prostate volume demonstrated a statistically significant association with csPC (Table 4).

Table 3. Association between clinically significant prostate cancer (csPC) diagnosis and other factors, digital rectal examination (DRE) excluded.

	MVA vs. csPC OR (95% CI), *p*-Value
Age, years	1.05 (1.03–1.08), <0.001
Biopsy-naïve	1.69 (1.17–2.44), 0.005
PSA > 10 ng/mL	2.43 (1.58–3.75), <0.001
PV, mL	0.98 (0.97–0.98), <0.001
Max. lesion size, mm	1.06 (1.03–1.09), <0.001
PIRADS > 3	3.27 (1.69–6.31), <0.001
Lesion in PZ	1.95 (1.30–2.92), 0.001

MVA, multivariable analysis (logistic regression model, n = 697); OR, odds ratio; CI, confidence interval; PSA, prostate-specific antigen; PIRADS, prostate imaging reporting, and data system; PZ, peripheral zone; DRE, digital rectal examination.

Table 4. Association between clinically significant prostate cancer (csPC) diagnosis and other factors in patients with the highest PIRADS category 3.

	MVA vs. csPC, DRE Included OR (95% CI), *p*-Value	MVA vs. csPC, DRE Excluded OR (95% CI), *p*-Value
Age, years	1.08 (0.98–1.19), NS	1.08 (0.98–1.19), NS
Biopsy-naïve	0.81 (0.20–3.39), NS	0.86 (0.21–3.43), NS
PSA > 10 ng/mL	1.69 (0.32–8.86), NS	1.46 (0.28–7.52), NS
PV, mL	0.94 (0.90–0.99), 0.019	0.94 (0.89–0.99), 0.017
Max. lesion size, mm	1.02 (0.88–1.19), NS	1.03 (0.88–1.19), NS
Lesion in PZ	3.17 (0.58–17.37), NS	3.09 (0.58–16.34), NS
Positive DRE	2.93 (0.42–20.31), NS	N.A.

MVA, multivariable analysis (logistic regression model, n = 114); OR, odds ratio; CI, confidence interval; PSA, prostate specific antigen; PIRADS, prostate imaging reporting and data system; PZ, peripheral zone; DRE, digital rectal examination; NS—nonsignificant; N.A.—not-applicable.

4. Discussion

We present one of the largest series of MRI-positive patients who underwent biopsies of the prostate. MRI-ultrasound fusion biopsy was performed in every case, and while any possible superiority of this technique over cognitive biopsy remains controversial, with trends toward improved CDRs remaining statistically insignificant in a meta-analysis [8], fusion biopsy may serve as an acceptable reference standard in terms of evaluating MRI diagnostic values. We consider this a strength of our study.

Interestingly, our cancer detection rates, especially for PIRADS categories 4 and 5, were significantly lower than the available data would suggest. In a meta-analysis by Mazzone et al., rates of csPC with PIRADS categories 4 and 5 were reported to be 40% (95% CI: 34–46%) and 69% (65–73%), respectively [7], which barely overlaps with our 95% CIs for these values. Oerther et al., in a meta-analysis limited to studies in which PIRADS v. 2.1 was adopted, demonstrated the CDRs to be even higher [9]. The large heterogeneity between studies reporting CDRs in MRI-positive patients undergoing prostate biopsy is a well-recognized issue [7]. We believe that the most probable explanation for the relatively low rate of csPC in our patients is the significant (44%) proportion of men with a prior biopsy history. As demonstrated in the results, these men were significantly less likely to be diagnosed with csPC than biopsy-naïve patients, which is in accordance with available evidence. A recent prospective study by Patel et al. [10] also demonstrated that being biopsy-naïve was a significant factor for csPC diagnosis in MRI-positive patients, which confirms the trends previously described in the literature [7].

Given the abovementioned discrepancies in reported CDRs between cohorts of MRI-positive patients, the role of factors other than the PIRADS category in altering the probability of a csPC diagnosis is unquestionable, and our aim was to provide evidence regarding these associations. Being biopsy-naïve has already been discussed above. Age was another predictor we evaluated. While Washino et al. demonstrated no significant association between age and csPC in their patients [11], most studies report older age to be a strong predictor of csPC diagnosis, independently of the PIRADS category [10,12]. Whether this finding represents the well-established association between older age and increased incidence of csPC [13] or age-related features possibly altering MRI interpretation [14], remains beyond the scope of these considerations.

Given that non-csPC may not lead to PSA level elevations independent of the contribution of benign prostate tissue [15], high PSA levels should serve as predictors of csPC. Several studies demonstrated that PSA density (PSAD) may increase the risk of csPC independently of PIRADS category [10,11,16]. We decided to analyze PSA and PV as separate predictors, considering the possible independent association between smaller PV and csPC [17,18]. On multivariable analyses, we demonstrated significant associations with csPC for both PSA > 10 ng/mL and smaller PV. Moreover, in PIRADS category 3 patients, only the smaller PV was associated with higher csPC rates. To our knowledge, this is the first study in which PV was considered an independent risk factor in a regression model. Our results suggest that the relationship between those parameters and prostate cancer biology may be much more complex than represented by a proportion (i.e., PSAD). Further studies are needed to provide deeper insight into the predictive values of PSA and PV in patients suspected of harboring csPC.

We demonstrated that a larger maximum lesion size was associated with a higher CDR. In analyses performed on the overall group, this larger maximum lesion size might have represented a higher PIRADS category, given that $\geq$15 mm in the maximal dimension of a lesion is a criterion for assigning PIRADS category 5 instead of 4. Furthermore, in the analysis limited to PIRADS category 3 patients, the association between maximum lesion size and csPC was non-significant. Given the low CDR in this subgroup of patients, a small sample size might have been a limitation. Nevertheless, Tan et al., in a study on men who underwent in-bore MRI-guided transrectal targeted prostate biopsy, demonstrated no significant difference in the median diameter of the lesion between patients with negative and positive biopsy findings [19]. The role of maximum lesion size, other than differentiating between PIRADS categories 4 and 5, in stratifying the risk of csPC in men with positive MRIs should be subject to further studies.

Available data suggests that the prostate zone may serve as an additional factor predictive of csPS in patients with a positive MRI [20]. In the overall group, we demonstrated that a lesion located in the PZ was strongly associated with a higher CDR. In the PIRADS category three subgroup, despite a high OR, the association was non-significant, possibly due to an insufficient sample size. However, Kim et al., in a study on PIRADS category three patients who underwent MRI-ultrasound fusion targeted biopsy, did demonstrate that PZ location was an independent predictor of csPC [21]. Felker et al. suggested that many men with PIRADS category 3 lesions in the transition zone (TZ) might not be considered candidates for biopsy due to low csPC probability [22]. Our results may serve as additional evidence helpful in the decision-making process for these patients.

Despite multiple limitations, DRE remains a simple and cost-effective tool in the initial assessment of patients suspected of PC. While offering a biopsy of the prostate based solely on a positive DRE may be considered controversial in many cases, the available evidence proves that a positive DRE is a very strong predictor of csPC in MRI-positive patients. Chang et al. demonstrated that positive DRE had 91% specificity for csPC in men with positive MRI and elevated PSA who underwent MRI-ultrasound fusion biopsy [23]. Omri et al. also reported higher CDR in men with positive DRE [24]. In our study group, based on the results of multivariable analysis, patients with a positive DRE had almost double the odds of being diagnosed with csPC. The association in the PIRADS category 3 subgroup was non-significant. Nevertheless, both the literature data and our results demonstrate that a biopsy of the prostate should be offered to every man with an MRI and DRE suggestive of a malignant tumor.

We decided to perform separate analyses in the subgroup of PIRADS category 3 patients, as the low CDR in these men encourages the identification of risk factors, allowing for the offering of a prostate biopsy only to patients with a significant probability of a csPC diagnosis. In the study by Kim et al., older age, PZ location, and higher PSAD were associated with csPC on multivariable analysis [21]. Sheridan et al. demonstrated older age, smaller PV, and positive DRE as risk factors for csPC in patients with PIRADS category 3 lesions [25]. Felker et al. suggested PSAD $\geq$ 0.15 ng/mL^2 and an apparent diffusion coefficient (ADC) < 1000 mm^2/s as criteria that would lead to a much higher yield for csPC in men with PIRADS category 3 TZ lesions [22]. Recently, Schoots et al., based on the results of a meta-analysis that included data from 3006 biopsy-naïve patients, suggested that a prostate biopsy should be performed in a patient with a PIRADS category 3 lesion in the case of a PSAD $\geq$ 0.1 [26]. In our study, we managed to demonstrate a significant association only for smaller PV. The non-significance of other factors may be explained both by a lack of association and by the small sample size discussed above. Further studies on large populations or meta-analyses of available data are paramount to establishing the best evidence-based strategies for men with PIRADS category 3 lesions.

While we are aware that the discussed risk factors for detection of csPC have already been evaluated in the literature, this is the first large-volume study using MRI-ultrasound fusion biopsy results as a reference in which this particular set of clinically relevant and easily assessed factors was incorporated into a regression model. Hence, our results may possibly serve as evidence useful for weighted clinical judgment in patients in whom the individual low probability of harboring csPC is considered against the risk of biopsy complications. In our study, we adopted a per-patient, not per-lesion strategy for data analysis. The meta-analysis by Mazzone et al. demonstrated that per-lesion-level analysis may lead to lower rates of csPC [7]. Even with the use of a reference MRI-ultrasound fusion technique, cores still may miss the malignant lesion due to technical targeting mistakes or MRI limitations in detecting multifocal disease, and the identification of men who would benefit from omitting systematic cores is currently infeasible [27]. The per-patient study design was aimed to represent a typical clinical scenario.

While the multicenter design of the study may be considered a strength, some possible limitations must be addressed. All the biopsies were performed using the same software and materials. Hence, we deemed the quality of the cores to be similar between the centers. While the significantly lower median number of cores taken at Center 3 (Table 1) may raise concerns, this did not translate into decreased CDR in this institution. Although all the specimens were assessed according to the ISUP guidelines, possible interobserver variability between institutional pathologists might have been a source of bias. No uniform review of specimens may be considered a limitation of the study. Additionally, the results of DRE might have varied largely between the clinicians performing a biopsy. However, in order to exclude a possible bias caused by heterogeneity with regard to DRE interpretation, we performed a sub-analysis of the data without including DRE results.

Combining patients who underwent transrectal and transperineal biopsy into one cohort may be considered a possible cause of bias, as the non-inferiority of the transrectal approach in terms of csPC detection is not well-established [28]. However, in our patients, the difference in CDRs between transrectal and transperineal cases was non-significant. The main limitation of our study is its retrospective design, which implies several drawbacks. The study is prone to selection bias, as we were unable to verify uniform criteria for patients being referred to biopsy, which might have been at the discretion of various external urologists, and depending on the individual clinical judgment of each external urologist, some patients at the same risk might have been offered different diagnostic strategies. There was no standardized biopsy protocol used for our patients, which could have significantly influenced the pathologic outcomes. We lack data in regard to the number of targeted versus systematic cores, which could be valuable in the analyses. Considering the possibly important role of a second opinion [29], no uniform review of MRI scans poses the study at risk of bias due to potential initial misinterpretations. Some data gaps might have been a source of bias. Nevertheless, patients without sufficient data were not included in the regression models. Including follow-up data in the study, especially in regard to possible re-biopsy or radical prostatectomy specimens, could also have influenced the diagnostic performance of the pre-biopsy MRI. In addition, analysis of several other factors, like family history, multifocality, or anatomic lesion location (base vs. mid-prostate vs. apex), could have provided deeper insight into the heterogeneity of CDR in MRI-positive patients.

5. Conclusions

Our large, multicenter, retrospective study exploring the csPC detection rates in MRI-positive patients undergoing MRI-ultrasound fusion biopsy of the prostate provides new data regarding the predictive values of particular PIRADS categories, with our values being slightly lower than the current literature would suggest. This study serves as another piece of evidence that the probability of a csPC diagnosis in patients with the PIRADS 3 category is substantially low, warranting further risk stratification prior to offering a biopsy.

We managed to investigate several factors that further increase the probability of a csPC diagnosis in patients with a positive MRI. Apart from a higher PIRADS category or lesion size, patients were more likely to be diagnosed with csPC in cases of older age, lower PV, positive DRE, a lesion located in the PZ, and being biopsy-naïve. The role of lower PV was especially significant in PIRADS category 3 patients. The results of this study may be helpful in the decision-making process for patients considered for prostate biopsy. Moreover, they point to important future research directions.

Author Contributions: Conceptualization, S.S. and H.K.; methodology, S.S., H.K. and M.D.; software, M.D.; validation, H.K. and M.D.; formal analysis, M.D.; investigation, S.S., H.K., B.Z., M.M., M.Z. and A.T.; resources, S.S.; data curation, H.K. and M.D.; writing—original draft preparation, H.K.; writing—review and editing, S.S., H.K., M.D., R.S. and S.P.; visualization, H.K. and A.T.; supervision, P.K. and Ł.N.; project administration, P.K. and Ł.N. All authors have read and agreed to the published version of the manuscript.

Funding: This research received no external funding.

Institutional Review Board Statement: Not applicable.

Informed Consent Statement: Patient consent was waived due to the retrospective and noninterventional character of the study.

Data Availability Statement: The data analyzed in this study are available upon request from the corresponding author.

Conflicts of Interest: The authors declare no conflict of interest.

References

1. Rawla, P. Epidemiology of prostate cancer. *World J. Oncol.* **2019**, *10*, 63–89. [CrossRef] [PubMed]
2. Wang, L.; Lu, B.; He, M.; Wang, Y.; Wang, Z.; Du, L. Prostate Cancer Incidence and Mortality: Global Status and Temporal Trends in 89 Countries From 2000 to 2019. *Front. Public Health* **2022**, *10*, 811044. [CrossRef] [PubMed]
3. Butler, S.S.; Muralidhar, V.; Zhao, S.G.; Sanford, N.N.; Franco, I.; Fullerton, Z.H.; Chavez, J.; D'Amico, A.V.; Feng, F.Y.; Rebbeck, T.R.; et al. Prostate cancer incidence across stage, NCCN risk groups, and age before and after USPSTF Grade D recommendations against prostate-specific antigen screening in 2012. *Cancer* **2020**, *126*, 717–724. [CrossRef] [PubMed]
4. Padhani, A.R.; Weinreb, J.; Rosenkrantz, A.B.; Villeirs, G.; Turkbey, B.; Barentsz, J. Prostate Imaging-Reporting and Data System Steering Committee: PI-RADS v2 Status Update and Future Directions. *Eur. Urol.* **2019**, *75*, 385–396. [CrossRef] [PubMed]
5. Borghesi, M.; Bianchi, L.; Barbaresi, U.; Vagnoni, V.; Corcioni, B.; Gaudiano, C.; Fiorentino, M.; Giunchi, F.; Chessa, F.; Garofalo, M.; et al. Diagnostic performance of MRI/TRUS fusion-guided biopsies vs. systematic prostate biopsies in biopsy-naïve, previous negative biopsy patients and men undergoing active surveillance. *Minerva Urol. Nephrol.* **2021**, *73*, 357–366. [CrossRef]
6. European Association of Urology. EAU Guidelines. In Proceedings of the 2022 EAU Annual Congress, Amsterdam, The Netherlands, 1–4 July 2022; Available online: https://uroweb.org/guidelines/prostate-cancer/chapter/citation-information (accessed on 3 October 2022).
7. Mazzone, E.; Stabile, A.; Pellegrino, F.; Basile, G.; Cignoli, D.; Cirulli, G.O.; Sorce, G.; Barletta, F.; Scuderi, S.; Bravi, C.A.; et al. Positive Predictive Value of Prostate Imaging Reporting and Data System Version 2 for the Detection of Clinically Significant Prostate Cancer: A Systematic Review and Meta-analysis. *Eur. Urol. Oncol.* **2021**, *4*, 697–713. [CrossRef]
8. Watts, K.L.; Frechette, L.; Muller, B.; Ilinksy, D.; Kovac, E.; Sankin, A.; Aboumohamed, A. Systematic review and meta-analysis comparing cognitive vs. image-guided fusion prostate biopsy for the detection of prostate cancer. *Urol. Oncol. Semin. Orig. Investig.* **2020**, *38*, 734.e19–734.e25. [CrossRef]

9. Oerther, B.; Engel, H.; Bamberg, F.; Sigle, A.; Gratzke, C.; Benndorf, M. Cancer detection rates of the PI-RADSv2.1 assessment categories: Systematic review and meta-analysis on lesion level and patient level. *Prostate Cancer Prostatic Dis.* **2022**, *25*, 256–263. [CrossRef]
10. Patel, H.D.; Koehne, E.L.; Shea, S.M.; Bhanji, Y.; Gerena, M.; Gorbonos, A.; Quek, M.L.; Flanigan, R.C.; Goldberg, A.; Gupta, G.N. Risk of prostate cancer for men with prior negative biopsies undergoing magnetic resonance imaging compared with biopsy-naive men: A prospective evaluation of the PLUM cohort. *Cancer* **2022**, *128*, 75–84. [CrossRef]
11. Washino, S.; Okochi, T.; Saito, K.; Konishi, T.; Hirai, M.; Kobayashi, Y.; Miyagawa, T. Combination of prostate imaging reporting and data system (PI-RADS) score and prostate-specific antigen (PSA) density predicts biopsy outcome in prostate biopsy naïve patients. *BJU Int.* **2017**, *119*, 225–233. [CrossRef]
12 Radtke, J.P.; Wiesenfarth, M.; Kesch, C.; Freitag, M.T.; Alt, C.D.; Celik, K.; Distler, F.; Roth, W.; Wieczorek, K.; Stock, C.; et al. Combined Clinical Parameters and Multiparametric Magnetic Resonance Imaging for Advanced Risk Modeling of Prostate Cancer—Patient-tailored Risk Stratification Can Reduce Unnecessary Biopsies. *Eur. Urol.* **2017**, *72*, 888–896. [CrossRef] [PubMed]
13. Huynh-Le, M.-P.; Myklebust, T.Å.; Feng, C.H.; Karunamuni, R.; Johannesen, T.B.; Dale, A.M.; Andreassen, O.A.; Seibert, T.M. Age dependence of modern clinical risk groups for localized prostate cancer—A population-based study. *Cancer* **2020**, *126*, 1691–1699. [CrossRef] [PubMed]
14. Zhang, J.; Tian, W.-Z.; Hu, C.-H.; Niu, T.-L.; Wang, X.-L.; Chen, X.-Y. Age-related changes of normal prostate: Evaluation by MR diffusion tensor imaging. *Int. J. Clin. Exp. Med.* **2015**, *8*, 11220–11224. [PubMed]
15. Palsdottir, T.; Nordström, T.; Aly, M.; Lindberg, J.; Clements, M.; Egevad, L.; Grönberg, H.; Eklund, M. Are Prostate Specific-Antigen (PSA) and age associated with the risk of ISUP Grade 1 prostate cancer? Results from 72 996 individual biopsy cores in 6 083 men from the Stockholm3 study. *PLoS ONE* **2019**, *14*, e0218280. [CrossRef]
16. Stevens, E.; Truong, M.; Bullen, J.A.; Ward, R.D.; Purysko, A.S.; Klein, E.A. Clinical utility of PSAD combined with PI-RADS category for the detection of clinically significant prostate cancer. *Urol. Oncol. Semin. Orig. Investig.* **2020**, *38*, 846.e9–846.e16. [CrossRef]
17. Hong, S.K.; Poon, B.Y.; Sjoberg, D.D.; Scardino, P.T.; Eastham, J.A. Prostate Size and Adverse Pathologic Features in Men Undergoing Radical Prostatectomy. *Urology* **2014**, *84*, 153–157. [CrossRef]
18. Al-Khalil, S.; Ibilibor, C.; Cammack, J.T.; de Riese, W. Association of prostate volume with incidence and aggressiveness of prostate cancer. *Res. Rep. Urol.* **2016**, *8*, 201–205. [CrossRef]
19. Tan, N.; Lin, W.-C.; Khoshnoodi, P.; Asvadi, N.H.; Yoshida, J.; Margolis, D.J.A.; Lu, D.S.K.; Wu, H.; Sung, K.H.; Huang, J.; et al. In-Bore 3-T MR-guided Transrectal Targeted Prostate Biopsy: Prostate Imaging Reporting and Data System Version 2–based Diagnostic Performance for Detection of Prostate Cancer. *Radiology* **2017**, *283*, 130–139. [CrossRef]
20. Syed, J.S.; Nguyen, K.A.; Nawaf, C.B.; Bhagat, A.M.; Huber, S.; Levi, A.; Humphrey, P.; Weinreb, J.C.; Schulam, P.G.; Sprenkle, P.C. Prostate zonal anatomy correlates with the detection of prostate cancer on multiparametric magnetic resonance imaging/ultrasound fusion-targeted biopsy in patients with a solitary PI-RADS v2-scored lesion. *Urol. Oncol.* **2017**, *35*, 542.e19–542.e24. [CrossRef]
21. Kim, T.J.; Lee, M.S.; Hwang, S.I.; Lee, H.J.; Hong, S.K. Outcomes of magnetic resonance imaging fusion-targeted biopsy of prostate imaging reporting and data system 3 lesions. *World J. Urol.* **2018**, *37*, 1581–1586. [CrossRef]
22. Felker, E.R.; Raman, S.S.; Margolis, D.J.; Lu, D.S.K.; Shaheen, N.; Natarajan, S.; Sharma, D.; Huang, J.; Dorey, F.; Marks, L.S. Risk stratification among men with Prostate Imaging Reporting and Data System version 2 category 3 transition zone lesions: Is biopsy always necessary? *Am. J. Roentgenol.* **2017**, *209*, 1272–1277. [CrossRef] [PubMed]
23. Chang, C.M.; McIntosh, A.G.; Shapiro, D.D.; Davis, J.W.; Ward, J.F.; Gregg, J.R. Does a screening digital rectal exam provide actionable clinical utility in patients with an elevated PSA and positive MRI? *BJUI Compass* **2021**, *2*, 188–193. [CrossRef] [PubMed]
24. Omri, N.; Alex, S.; Jacob, B.; Ofer, N. The additive value of mpMRI on prostate cancer detection: Comparison between patients with and without a suspicious digital rectal examination (DRE). *Urol. Oncol. Semin. Orig. Investig.* **2021**, *39*, 728.e7–728.e11. [CrossRef] [PubMed]
25. Sheridan, A.D.; Nath, S.K.; Syed, J.S.; Aneja, S.; Sprenkle, P.C.; Weinreb, J.C.; Spektor, M. Risk of Clinically Significant Prostate Cancer Associated With Prostate Imaging Reporting and Data System Category 3 (Equivocal) Lesions Identified on Multiparametric Prostate MRI. *Am. J. Roentgenol.* **2018**, *210*, 347–357. [CrossRef]
26. Schoots, I.G.; Padhani, A.R. Risk-adapted biopsy decision based on prostate magnetic resonance imaging and prostate-specific antigen density for enhanced biopsy avoidance in first prostate cancer diagnostic evaluation. *Br. J. Urol.* **2021**, *127*, 175–178. [CrossRef]
27. Dell'Oglio, P.; Stabile, A.; Soligo, M.; Brembilla, G.; Esposito, A.; Gandaglia, G.; Fossati, N.; Bravi, C.A.; Dehò, F.; De Cobelli, F.; et al. There Is No Way to Avoid Systematic Prostate Biopsies in Addition to Multiparametric Magnetic Resonance Imaging Targeted Biopsies. *Eur. Urol. Oncol.* **2020**, *3*, 112–118. [CrossRef]
28. Xiang, J.; Yan, H.; Li, J.; Wang, X.; Chen, H.; Zheng, X. Transperineal versus transrectal prostate biopsy in the diagnosis of prostate cancer: A systematic review and meta-analysis. *World J. Surg. Oncol.* **2019**, *17*, 31. [CrossRef]

29. Luzzago, S.; Petralia, G.; Musi, G.; Catellani, M.; Alessi, S.; Di Trapani, E.; Mistretta, F.; Serino, A.; Conti, A.; Pricolo, P.; et al. Multiparametric Magnetic Resonance Imaging Second Opinion May Reduce the Number of Unnecessary Prostate Biopsies: Time to Improve Radiologists' Training Program? *Clin. Genitourin. Cancer* **2019**, *17*, 88–96. [CrossRef]

Journal of
Clinical Medicine

MDPI

Article

Nomograms Combining PHI and PI-RADS in Detecting Prostate Cancer: A Multicenter Prospective Study

Yongheng Zhou [1,†], Qiang Fu [2,†], Zhiqiang Shao [3,†], Keqin Zhang [2], Wenqiang Qi [1], Shangzhen Geng [1], Wenfu Wang [1], Jianfeng Cui [1], Xin Jiang [1], Rongyang Li [4], Yaofeng Zhu [1,*], Shouzhen Chen [1,*] and Benkang Shi [1,*]

1 Department of Urology, Qilu Hospital of Shandong University, Jinan 250012, China
2 Department of Urology, Shandong Provincial Hospital, Jinan 250000, China
3 Department of Urology, Linyi People's Hospital, Linyi 276000, China
4 Department of Thoracic Surgery, Qilu Hospital of Shandong University, Jinan 250012, China
* Correspondence: feng2209@email.sdu.edu.cn (Y.Z.); chenshouzhen@email.sdu.edu.cn (S.C.); bkang68@sdu.edu.cn (B.S.)
† These authors contributed equally to this work.

Abstract: (1) Background: The study aimed to construct nomograms to improve the detection rates of prostate cancer (PCa) and clinically significant prostate cancer (CSPCa) in the Asian population. (2) Methods: This multicenter prospective study included a group of 293 patients from three hospitals. Univariable and multivariable logistic regression analysis was performed to identify potential risk factors and construct nomograms. Discrimination, calibration, and clinical utility were used to assess the performance of the nomogram. The web-based dynamic nomograms were subsequently built based on multivariable logistic analysis. (3) Results: A total of 293 patients were included in our study with 201 negative and 92 positive results in PCa. Four independent predictive factors (age, prostate health index (PHI), prostate volume, and prostate imaging reporting and data system score (PI-RADS)) for PCa were included, and four factors (age, PHI, PI-RADS, and Log PSA Density) for CSPCa were included. The area under the ROC curve (AUC) for PCa was 0.902 in the training cohort and 0.869 in the validation cohort. The AUC for CSPCa was 0.896 in the training cohort and 0.890 in the validation cohort. (4) Conclusions: The combined diagnosis of PHI and PI-RADS can avoid more unnecessary biopsies and improve the detection rate of PCa and CSPCa. The nomogram with the combination of age, PHI, PV, and PI-RADS could improve the detection of PCa, and the nomogram with the combination of age, PHI, PI-RADS, and Log PSAD could improve the detection of CSPCa.

Keywords: multiparametric magnetic resonance imaging; prostate health index; prostate cancer; nomogram; diagnosis

1. Introduction

Globally, prostate cancer (PCa) is the second leading cause of death among men, with approximately 268,490 new cases and 34,500 deaths projected to occur in America by 2022. [1]. With the widespread use of prostate-specific antigen (PSA), the early diagnosis and treatment of PCa are gradually increasing [2]. However, the low specificity of PSA has led to lots of unnecessary and excessive prostate biopsies, resulting in a significant financial burden as well as many post-biopsy complications. In recent years, scholars have used different biomarkers, such as the 4Kscore, PCA3, and the prostate health index (PHI), and different predictive models to improve the detection rate of prostate cancer [3–5]. The clinical application of prostate multiparametric magnetic resonance imaging (mpMRI) and the prostate imaging reporting and data system (PI-RADS) has also improved the diagnosis of PCa and clinically significant prostate cancer (CSPCa) in terms of imaging [6]. With the combination of the above biomarkers with mpMRI, cancer detection rates have been improved and unnecessary biopsies have been reduced [7].

The discovery and clinical application of (-2) proPSA (P2PSA) have made PHI an important indicator for low-risk and intermediate-risk PCa screening, especially in PSA 2–20 ng/mL, in clinical practice [8,9]. A large cohort study showed that a cutoff value of 35 for PHI in Asian populations reached good sensitivity and specificity [8]. However, in actual clinical work, it is insufficient to use the PHI value of 35 as a cutoff value for diagnosing prostate cancer. Therefore, the role of the combined diagnosis of PCa appears to be important.

The purpose of this study is to construct clinically useful nomograms using PHI and PI-RADS indicators, along with other clinical indicators, which are based on data from a multicenter database, in order to improve the diagnostic accuracy of PCa and CSPCa in the Asian population.

2. Materials and Methods

2.1. Study Population

This multicenter prospective study included a group of 293 patients from three hospitals in the Asian population, 29 patients from hospital 1, 42 patients from hospital 2, and 222 patients from hospital 3. This study is a prospective multicenter observational cohort study and the clinical trial registration number is NCT05179707. It has been approved by the Ethics Committee of Qilu Hospital of Shandong University and endorsed by the Ethics Committees of the other institutions participating in the study. All patients signed a written informed consent form. Patients with PSA in 4–20 ng/mL and a normal digital rectal examination were enrolled. If a patient's mpMRI showed a low probability of cancer and a PSA level of around 4 ng/mL, we elaborated on different treatment options for the patient, including active surveillance and other treatment modalities. If the patient had a very strong desire for a biopsy, we performed a biopsy after that patient signed an informed consent form.

The exclusion criteria were as follows: (I) abnormal blood clotting function; (II) infection of the urinary tract or prostatitis; (III) prostate surgery (such as transurethral resection of the prostate) performed prior to biopsy. The patients in this cohort were all biopsy-naive.

2.2. Data Collection and Clinical Variables

Before prostate biopsy, blood samples were collected prospectively to determine total prostate-specific antigen (TPSA), free prostate-specific antigen (fPSA), and P2PSA levels. A blood clotting process was performed at room temperature for one hour, followed by centrifugation for fifteen minutes. A serum sample was aliquoted, frozen at −80 °C, and subjected to immunoassay using dedicated Access TPSA, fPSA, and P2PSA reagents (Beckman Coulter, Brea, CA, USA). Calculation of the f/T indicator was completed by dividing the fPSA by the TPSA, and calculation of the PSAD was performed by dividing the TPSA by the PV. These data were calculated using the prostate ellipsoid formulation: PV = ([maximum anteroposterior diameter] × [maximum transverse diameter] × [maximum longitudinal diameter] × 0.52], measured using an MRI scan [10]. Based on Beckman and Coulter's PHI formula, the PHI was calculated as follows: ((-2) proPSA/free PSA) / $\sqrt{}$PSA, and %P2PSA was calculated using the formula [(P2PSA pg/mL)/ (fPSA ng/mL × 1000)] × 100 [9,11].

A mpMRI was performed on all patients prior to prostate biopsy using a 3.0 T machine without an endorectal coil. The scanning protocol of mpMRI included T1-weighted imaging (T1WI), T2-weighted imaging (T2WI), diffusion-weighted imaging (DWI), and dynamic contrast-enhanced imaging (DCE). DWI was acquired with b values of 0 and 1500 s/mm^2, and an apparent diffusion coefficient (ADC) map was generated. The mpMRI was interpreted by two urogenital radiologists with at least three years of experience in prostate MRI and recorded by using the PI-RADS v2.1 score. There is a very low probability that CSPCa will be present in PI-RADS 1 (CSPCa is highly unlikely to occur); PI-RADS 2 (CSPCa is highly unlikely to occur); PI-RADS 3 (equivocal presence of CSPCa); PI-RADS 4—High (CSPCa is highly likely to occur); PI-RADS 5—Very high (CSPCa is highly likely to occur) [12,13].

All patients underwent ultrasound-guided transperineal prostate biopsy or transrectal prostate biopsy in antibiotic prophylaxis. The patients underwent 12-core systematic prostate biopsy and an additional 4-core biopsy was performed in suspicious lesions. MRI-transrectal/transperineal cognitive fusion biopsy was performed for the suspicious lesions. When using transperineal prostate biopsy, physicians use a free-hand approach biopsy. Biopsies were performed at each center by physicians with at least five years of experience in biopsy procedures. According to the guidelines of the International Society of Urological Pathology Consensus Conference, biopsy specimens were interpreted and graded [14]. PCa was defined as Gleason score (GS) $\geq 3 + 3$ and CSPCa was defined as GS $\geq 3 + 4$ [15].

2.3. Construction of the PCa and CSPCa Nomograms

The entire cohort was randomly divided into a training cohort and a validation cohort in a 3:1 ratio, and we used the training cohort to build the nomogram and the validation cohort for verification. The potential risk factors for PCa and CSPCa were identified using a univariable logistic regression analysis. The factors with a P value less than 0.1 in univariable logistic regression analysis were included in the multivariable logistic regression analysis. The final predictive models using the independent risk factors ($p < 0.05$ in multivariable stepwise forward logistic regression) were constructed. Following the multivariable logistic regression analysis, nomograms were constructed using the R packages "rms" and "DynNom" (version 4.1.1; http://www.r-project.org/, 3 August 2022). Using the regression model, scores were calculated for each variable, and the predicted probability of PCa and CSPCa was determined by averaging the scores.

2.4. Nomogram Performance

In order to evaluate the performance of the nomogram, discrimination, calibration, and clinical utility were taken into account. Discrimination consists of evaluating a model for its ability to distinguish between events and non-events. An evaluation of the predictive nomogram's discrimination efficiency was conducted using a receiver operating characteristic (ROC) curve [16]. A calibration process was used to determine the degree to which predicted probabilities correspond to actual results. The calibration power was assessed using the Hosmer–Lemeshow test, and a P value greater than 0.05 was considered satisfactory. A bootstrapping method with 1000 replications was used for internal validation [17]. Evaluation of clinical utility was conducted using decision curve analysis (DCA).

2.5. Statistical Analysis

For the comparison of the continuous variables of groups, the normality test was first performed, and the Student t-test was used for continuous variables that met the normality test; otherwise, the Mann–Whitney U test was applied for continuous variables. Normally distributed continuous variables were described as mean $\pm$ standard deviation (SD); otherwise, the form of the median (interquartile range (IQR)) was described. Ranked data were analyzed by using the Wilcoxon rank sum test. The Kruskall Wallis test was used to analyze the variables between multiple groups. Some indicators with over-inflated odds ratio (OR) values were balanced using Log transformation. The optimal cut-off value of the nomogram was obtained from the maximum Youden index. p value < 0.05 was considered statistically significant. Data analysis was conducted using R Project software (version 4.1.1; http://www.R-project.org, 3 August 2022) and SPSS software (version 25.0; SPSS Inc., Chicago, IL, USA).

3. Results

A total of 293 patients were included in our study with 201 negative and 92 positive results in PCa between September 2020 to June 2022. A comparison of the baseline demographic characteristics from the three hospitals is shown in Table S1. In the cohort, patients were randomly assigned to the training cohort (n = 220) or the validation cohort (n = 73). No significant differences were observed in any of the variables between the two cohorts

(Table 1). The characteristics of patients in the training and validation cohorts are shown in Tables 2 and 3.

Table 1. Patients' characteristics of the training cohort and validation cohort in total and significant prostate cancer.

Characteristics	All Cohort	PCa			CSPCa		
		Training Cohort	Validation Cohort	p Value	Training Cohort	Validation Cohort	p Value
N (%)	293 (100)	220 (75.09)	73 (24.91)	-	220 (75.09)	73 (24.91)	-
Age (years), median (IQR)	66.00 (60.00–72.00)	66.00 (59.25–72.75)	66.00 (61.00–72.00)	0.787	66.00 (60.00–72.00)	66.00 (60.00–74.00)	0.355
TPSA (ng/mL), median (IQR)	8.51 (5.97–12.11)	8.59 (5.96–12.13)	8.31 (5.95–11.93)	0.956	8.51 (5.88–11.96)	8.84 (6.11–12.99)	0.478
fPSA (ng/mL), median (IQR)	1.13 (0.79–1.61)	1.12 (0.79–1.60)	1.14 (0.76–1.73)	0.697	1.13 (0.75–1.60)	1.21 (0.91–1.67)	0.396
P2PSA (ng/mL), median (IQR)	17.89 (12.01–28.90)	17.97 (12.95–22.35)	17.89 (10.98–29.76)	0.783	17.83 (11.80–28.62)	20.54 (14.25–29.87)	0.226
PHI, median (IQR)	47.15 (35.36–67.90)	47.65 (35.18–67.91)	46.28 (35.16–68.51)	0.842	46.51 (25.09–69.60)	48.80 (37.42–63.95)	0.574
f/T, median (IQR)	0.14 (0.10–0.19)	0.14 (0.09–0.19)	0.13 (0.11–0.19)	0.690	0.14 (0.09–0.20)	0.14 (0.10–0.19)	0.679
%P2PSA, median (IQR)	1.70 (1.27–2.27)	1.71 (1.30–2.23)	1.70 (1.15–2.28)	0.955	1.69 (1.26–2.27)	1.73 (1.33–2.28)	0.582
PV (mL), median (IQR)	44.13 (28.84–65.54)	44.45 (28.84–66.23)	43.68 (28.53–63.86)	0.820	42.46 (28.22–63.10)	45.45 (31.43–67.27)	0.381
PI-RADS, n (%)				0.963			0.359
≤2	117 (39.9)	85 (38.6)	32 (43.8)		91 (41.4)	26 (35.6)	
3	92 (31.4)	76 (34.5)	16 (21.9)		69 (31.4)	23 (31.5)	
≥4	84 (28.7)	59 (26.8)	25 (34.2)		60 (27.3)	24 (32.9)	
PSAD (ng/mL^2), median (IQR)	0.19 (0.13–0.31)	0.18 (0.12–0.31)	0.21 (0.13–0.33)	0.589	0.18 (0.12–0.31)	0.21	0.871

IQR: interquartile range; TPSA: total prostate-specific antigen; fPSA: free prostate-specific antigen; P2PSA: (-2)pro-prostate-specific antigen; PHI: prostate health index; f/T: free/total prostate-specific antigen; %P2PSA: defined as [(P2PSA/fPSA) × 100]; PV: prostate volume; PI-RADS: Prostate Imaging-Reporting and Data System; PSAD: prostate-specific antigen density; CSPCa: clinically significant prostate cancer, defined as Gleason Grade ≥ 2. The P value is for comparing the training cohort with the validation cohort.

Table 2. Patient characteristics in training and validation cohorts with and without PCa.

Characteristics	Training Cohort			Validation Cohort		
	Non-PCa	PCa	p Value	Non-PCa	PCa	p Value
Age (years), median (IQR)	66.00 (59.00–71.50)	67.00 (64.00–74.00)	0.094	63.50 (58.00–69.75)	71.00 (66.00–77.00)	0.001
TPSA (ng/mL), median (IQR)	8.38 (5.57–11.59)	8.97 (6.38–13.58)	0.106	7.98 (5.65–10.48)	11.03 (7.14–13.69)	0.023
fPSA (ng/mL), median (IQR)	1.23 (0.81–1.70)	1.06 (0.79–1.39)	0.196	1.11 (0.85–1.69)	1.40 (0.74–1.78)	0.622
P2PSA (ng/mL), median (IQR)	16.57 (10.93–23.62)	25.57 (31.58–52.10)	0.000	15.20 (9.65–24.64)	30.44 (15.45–49.74)	0.001
PHI, median (IQR)	42.07 (31.58–52.10)	72.57 (51.67–110.15)	0.000	40.74 (28.62–53.92)	73.11 (59.45–98.91)	0.000
f/T, median (IQR)	0.15 (0.10–0.21)	0.12 (0.09–0.15)	0.001	0.14 (0.11–0.20)	0.13 (0.08–0.17)	0.338
%P2PSA, median (IQR)	1.47 (1.03–1.85)	2.44 (1.87–3.20)	0.000	1.58 (1.05–2.03)	2.30 (1.76–3.23)	0.000
PV (mL), median (IQR)	50.39 (35.03–73.81)	32.85 (23.06–47.67)	0.000	50.16 (32.90–66.55)	30.40 (20.14–48.64)	0.010

Table 2. *Cont.*

Characteristics	Training Cohort			Validation Cohort		
	Non-PCa	PCa	p Value	Non-PCa	PCa	p Value
PI-RADS, n (%)			0.000			0.002
≤2	77 (51.7)	8 (11.3)		29 (55.8)	3 (14.3)	
3	51 (34.2)	25 (35.2)		11 (21.2)	5 (23.8)	
≥4	21 (14.1)	38 (53.5)		12 (23.1)	13 (61.9)	
PSAD (ng/mL^2), median (IQR)	0.16 (0.11–0.24)	0.25 (0.18–0.47)	0.000	0.17 (0.11–0.25)	0.36 (0.23–0.43)	0.000

IQR: interquartile range; TPSA: total prostate-specific antigen; fPSA: free prostate-specific antigen; P2PSA: (-2)pro-prostate-specific antigen; PHI: prostate health index; f/T: free/total prostate-specific antigen; %P2PSA: defined as [(P2PSA/fPSA) × 100]; PV: prostate volume; PI-RADS: Prostate Imaging-Reporting and Data System; PSAD: prostate-specific antigen density; PCa: prostate cancer. P value is for the comparison between non-PCa and PCa in the training cohort and validation cohort, respectively.

Table 3. Patient characteristics in training and validation cohorts with and without CSPCa.

Characteristics	Training Cohort			Validation Cohort		
	Non-PCa	PCa	p Value	Non-PCa	PCa	p Value
Age (years), median (IQR)	66.00 (59.00–71.50)	67.00 (64.00–74.00)	0.094	63.50 (58.00–69.75)	71.00 (66.00–77.00)	0.001
TPSA (ng/mL), median (IQR)	8.38 (5.57–11.59)	8.97 (6.38–13.58)	0.106	7.98 (5.65–10.48)	11.03 (7.14–13.69)	0.023
fPSA (ng/mL), median (IQR)	1.23 (0.81–1.70)	1.06 (0.79–1.39)	0.196	1.11 (0.85–1.69)	1.40 (0.74–1.78)	0.622
P2PSA (ng/mL), median (IQR)	16.57 (10.93–23.62)	25.57 (31.58–52.10)	0.000	15.20 (9.65–24.64)	30.44 (15.45–49.74)	0.001
PHI, median (IQR)	42.07 (31.58–52.10)	72.57 (51.67–110.15)	0.000	40.74 (28.62–53.92)	73.11 (59.45–98.91)	0.000
f/T, median (IQR)	0.15 (0.10–0.21)	0.12 (0.09–0.15)	0.001	0.14 (0.11–0.20)	0.13 (0.08–0.17)	0.338
%P2PSA, median (IQR)	1.47 (1.03–1.85)	2.44 (1.87–3.20)	0.000	1.58 (1.05–2.03)	2.30 (1.76–3.23)	0.000
PV (mL), median (IQR)	50.39 (35.03–73.81)	32.85 (23.06–47.67)	0.000	50.16 (32.90–66.55)	30.40 (20.14–48.64)	0.010
PI-RADS, n (%)			0.000			0.002
≤2	77 (51.7)	8 (11.3)		29 (55.8)	3 (14.3)	
3	51 (34.2)	25 (35.2)		11 (21.2)	5 (23.8)	
≥4	21 (14.1)	38 (53.5)		12 (23.1)	13 (61.9)	
PSAD (ng/mL^2), median (IQR)	0.16 (0.11–0.24)	0.25 (0.18–0.47)	0.000	0.17 (0.11–0.25)	0.36 (0.23–0.43)	0.000

IQR: interquartile range; TPSA: total prostate-specific antigen; fPSA: free prostate-specific antigen; P2PSA: (-2)pro-prostate-specific antigen; PHI: prostate health index; f/T: free/total prostate-specific antigen; %P2PSA: defined as [(P2PSA/fPSA) × 100]; PV: prostate volume; PI-RADS: Prostate Imaging-Reporting and Data System; PSAD: prostate-specific antigen density; CSPCa: clinically significant prostate cancer, defined as Gleason Grade ≥ 2. P value is for the comparison between non-CSPCa and CSPCa in the training cohort and validation cohort, respectively.

3.1. Univariable and Multivariable Regression Analyses in Predicting PCa and CSPCa

An evaluation of the risk factors for PCa and CSPCa in the training cohort was conducted using both univariable and multivariable stepwise forward regression analyses (Table 4). Univariable logistic regression analyses showed that age, TPSA, P2PSA, PHI, f/T, %P2PSA, PV, PI-RADS, and Log (PSAD) were risk factors in predicting PCa and CSPCa. After analysis of the clinical value of the predictors and the collinearity, age, TPSA, PHI, f/T, PV, and PI-RADS were included into the multivariable regression analysis. Multivariable stepwise forward regression analysis revealed that age (OR = 0.970; 95% confidence interval (CI): 0.952–0.988; p = 0.014), PHI (OR = 1.037; 95% CI: 1.022–1.052; p = 0.000), PV (OR = 0.970; 95% CI: 0.952–0.988; p = 0.002), and PI-RADS (OR = 2.936; 95% CI: 1.873–4.601; p = 0.000) were predictive factors in detecting PCa. The risk factors for detecting CSPCa in multivariable regression analysis were PHI (OR = 1.033; 95% CI: 1.020–1.045; p = 0.000), Log (PSAD) (OR = 9.758; 95% CI: 2.458–39.220; p = 0.001), and PI-RADS (OR = 2.458; 95% CI: 1.709–3.535; p = 0.000).

Table 4. Univariable and multivariable logistic regression analysis of risk factors for total and significant prostate cancer in the training cohort.

Variable	PCa						CSPCa					
	Univariable Analysis			Multivariable Analysis			Univariable Analysis			Multivariable Analysis		
	OR	95% CI	*p* Value	OR	95% CI	*p* Value	OR	95% CI	*p* Value	OR	95% CI	*p* Value
Age	1.028	0.996–1.061	0.084	0.970	0.952–0.988	0.014	1.038	1.002–1.076	0.040			
TPSA	1.057	0.993–1.124	0.081				1.097	1.024–1.176	0.008			
fPSA	0.736	0.499–1.085	0.122				0.794	0.527–1.196	0.269			
P2PSA	1.045	1.025–1.066	0.000				1.047	1.026–1.068	0.000			
PHI	1.044	1.030–1.059	0.000	1.037	1.022–1.052	0.000	1.046	1.032–1.061	0.000	1.033	1.020–1.045	0.000
f/T	0.002	0.000–0.196	0.007				0.001	0.000–0.078	0.003			
%P2PSA	3.652	2.389–5.583	0.000				3.004	2.058–4.383	0.000			
PV	0.970	0.956–0.984	0.000	0.970	0.952–0.988	0.002	0.964	0.947–0.981	0.000			
PI-RADS	3.385	2.319–4.941	0.000	2.936	1.873–4.601	0.000	2.805	1.970–3.994	0.000	2.458	1.709–3.535	0.000
Log (PSAD)	22.300	6.809–73.042	0.000				72.227	16.817–310.206	0.000	9.758	2.458–39.220	0.001

TPSA: total prostate-specific antigen; fPSA: free prostate-specific antigen; P2PSA: (-2)pro-prostate-specific antigen; PHI: prostate health index; f/T: free/total prostate-specific antigen; %P2PSA: defined as [(P2PSA/fPSA) × 100]; PV: prostate volume; PI-RADS: Prostate Imaging-Reporting and Data System; PSAD: prostate-specific antigen density; PCa: prostate cancer; OR: odds ratio; CI: confidence interval. CSPCa: clinically significant prostate cancer, defined as Gleason Grade ≥ 2.

3.2. The Construction and Performance of Nomogram

Four independent predictive factors (age, PHI, PV, and PI-RADS) for PCa were included and four factors (age, PHI, PI-RADS, and Log PSAD) for CSPCa were included. Detailed information on the predictive model is shown in Table 5. The predictive models of PCa and CSPCa were constructed based on coefficients of the multivariable logistic regression model and are shown in Figure 1. There were totals of 7 axes in this nomogram, and 4 axes represented predictive factors. In order to calculate the estimated score for each risk factor, a perpendicular line can be drawn along the axis of the top points, and an additional sum can be computed to determine the total score. Additionally, we developed two web-based operation interfaces (https://zhouyonghengql.shinyapps.io/PCa_DynNom/) (https://zhouyonghengql.shinyapps.io/CSPCa_DynNomapp/) using the "Dynnom" package for urology surgeons in order to facilitate the widespread use of our predictive nomograms on 20 August 2022.

Table 5. Detailed information about the predictive model used to calculate the probability of PCa.

Risk Factors	Coefficient	SE	OR (95% CI)	*p*
PCa				
Intercept	−8.508	1.754	0.000	0.000
Age	0.058	0.024	0.970 (0.952–0.988)	0.014
PHI	0.036	0.008	1.037 (1.022–1.052)	0.000
PV	−0.030	0.010	0.970 (0.952–0.988)	0.002
PI-RADS	1.077	0.229	2.936 (1.873–4.601)	0.000
CSPCa				
Intercept	−5.341	1.717	0.005	0.002
Age	0.020	0.023	1.020 (0.975–1.067)	0.383
PHI	0.032	0.007	1.032 (1.018–1.047)	0.000
PI-RADS	0.850	0.217	2.340 (1.529–3.580)	0.000
Log (PASD)	2.515	0.835	12.370 (2.406–63.583)	0.003

PCa: prostate cancer; CSPCa: clinically significant prostate cancer, defined as Gleason Grade ≥ 2; SE: standard error; OR: odds ratio; CI: confidence interval. Probability of PCa in PSA 4–20 ng/mL can be calculated by using the following formula: ln (p/1-p) = 0.058 × Age + 0.036 × PHI-0.030 × PV + 1.077 × PI-RADS-8.508. Probability of CSPCa in PSA 4–20 ng/mL can be calculated by using the following formula: ln (p/1-p) = 0.020 × Age + 0.032 × PHI + 0.850 × PI-RADS + 2.515 × Log (PSAD)-5.341.

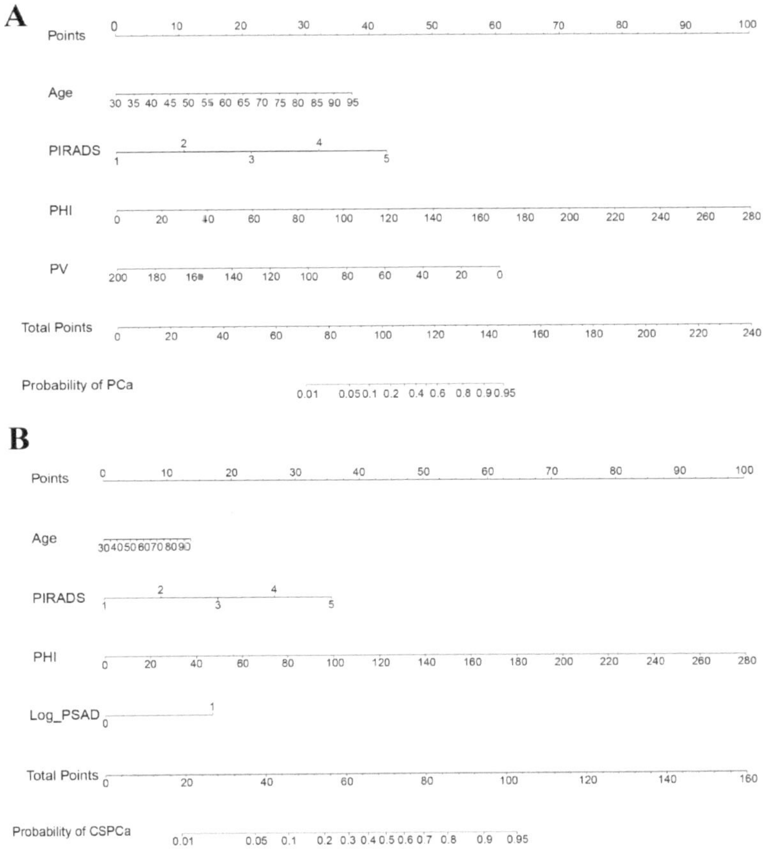

Figure 1. Nomograms for PCa (**A**) and CSPCa (**B**). In order to determine the point of each variable, draw a vertical line from the corresponding axis of the variable to the points axis. To estimate the probability of PCa/CSPCa, the total score can be projected to the lower total point axis by summing the points for each variable. PIRADS: Prostate Imaging-Reporting and Data System; PHI: prostate health index; PV: prostate volume; PSAD: prostate-specific antigen density; PCa: prostate cancer; CSPCa: clinically significant prostate cancer, defined as Gleason Grade ≥ 2.

The ROC curve was used to evaluate the accuracy of the predictive models and nomograms in discrimination capacity (Figure 2). The area under the ROC curve (AUC) for PCa was 0.9023 (95% CI: 0.8578–0.9467) in the training cohort and 0.8690 (95% CI: 0.7673–0.9707) in the validation cohort, which indicated that the nomogram had relatively high predictive accuracy. The optimal cut-off of the nomogram was 0.304, and the specificity and sensitivity were 0.841 and 0.859, respectively. In addition, the nomogram could avoid 57.68% of biopsies, and only 4.44% of patients with PCa were missed in this cut-off value.

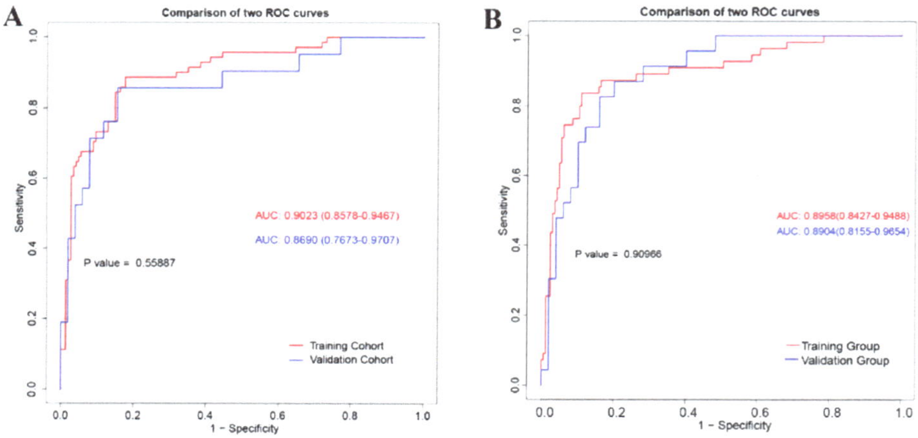

Figure 2. The receiver operating characteristic (ROC) curve of training cohort and validation cohort for PCa (**A**) and CSPCa (**B**). PCa: prostate cancer; CSPCa: clinically significant prostate cancer, defined as Gleason Grade ≥ 2; AUCs, areas under the ROC curve.

The Hosmer–Lemeshow test and calibration plot were used to assess calibration power. According to the Hosmer–Lemeshow test, the P value in the training cohort was 0.084 and, in the validation cohort, it was 0.397, indicating that the difference between the predicted probabilities and the actual probabilities was not significant. Both the training and validation cohort calibration plots (Figure 3) demonstrate that the predictive nomogram was well-calibrated. The DCA curve is shown in Figure S1.

The different cut-off values of PHI and the optimal cut-off values of nomograms are shown in Table 6. When the PHI value was greater than or equal to 35, the sensitivity and the specificity were 95.77% and 34.90%, respectively, and 23.64% of biopsies could be saved. When applying the nomogram for predicting PCa, 55.91% of biopsies could be saved, accompanied by 3.67% of PCa as well as 1.82% of CSPCa being missed.

Table 6. Predictive performance of different cut-off values of PHI and optimal cut-off values of nomograms.

	Sensitivity	Specificity	PPV	NPV	% Biopsy Avoided	% PCa Missed	%CSPCa Missed
PHI ≥ 35	95.77	34.90	41.21	94.55	23.64	1.36	1.36
PHI ≥ 40	90.14	45.64	44.14	90.67	30.91	3.18	1.82
PHI ≥ 45	81.69	59.73	49.15	87.25	40.45	5.91	3.18
PHI ≥ 50	76.06	71.81	56.25	86.29	48.64	7.73	4.09
PHI ≥ 55	74.65	79.87	63.86	86.86	54.09	8.18	4.55
[a] NP ≥ 27%	88.73	82.55	70.79	93.89	55.91	3.67	1.82
[b] NP ≥ 31%	83.64	89.09	71.88	94.23	63.64	7.27	4.09

NP: nomogram predictive; a: nomogram for predicting PCa; b: nomogram for predicting CSPCa; PPV: positive predictive value; NPV: negative predictive value; PCa: prostate cancer; CSPCa: clinically significant prostate cancer, defined as Gleason Grade ≥ 2.

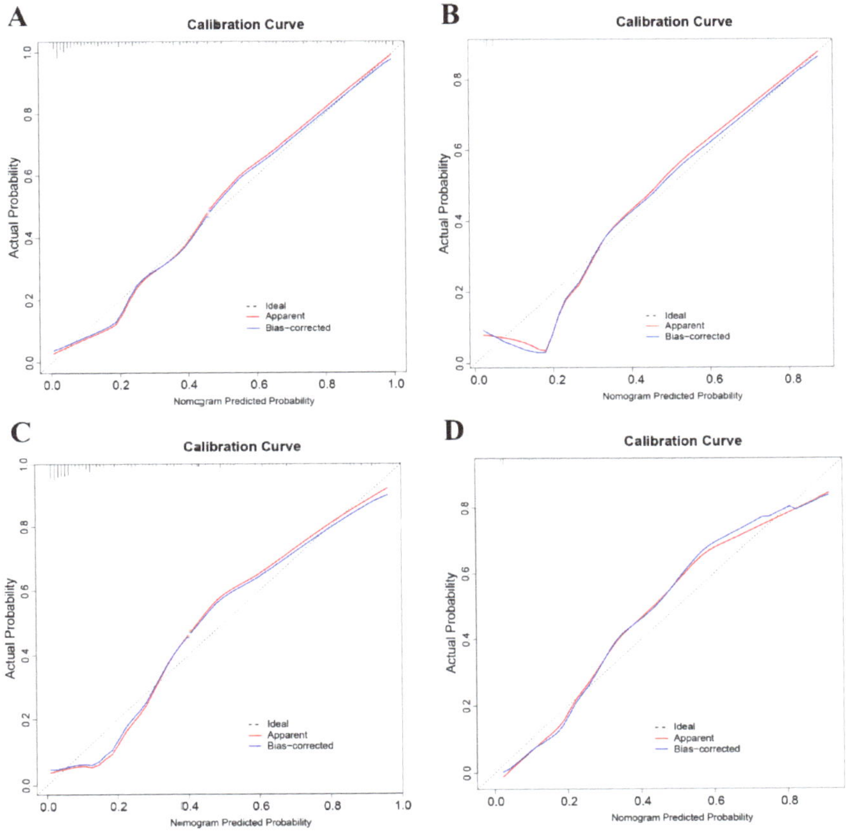

Figure 3. Prediction nomogram calibration curves for PCa in the training cohort (**A**) and validation cohort (**B**). The calibration curves for the CSPCa prediction nomogram in the training cohort (**C**) and validation cohort (**D**). On the x-axis, the nomogram-predicted probability is displayed, while on the y-axis, the actual probability of PCa or CSPCa is displayed. An ideal curve with a black point is represented by the black pointed line, an apparent curve with a red solid line represents the apparent curve that has not been corrected, and a bias-correction curve derived from bootstrapping (B = 1000 repetitions) is represented by the blue solid line. PCa: prostate cancer; CSPCa: clinically significant prostate cancer, defined as Gleason Grade ≥ 2.

4. Discussion

PCa is one of the common malignant tumors in men and prostate biopsy remains the gold standard for confirming PCa [18]. However, many patients experience unnecessary biopsies and suffer from the complications of biopsies. Therefore, the combined diagnosis of PCa has become quite important. Hsieh et al. found that the AUC of the combination of PHI and mpMRI (0.873 (95% CI 0.8050–0.9407)) was higher than the AUC of the PHI (0.735 (95% CI 0.6194–0.8497)) and the AUC of the mpMRI (0.830 (95% CI 0.7598–0.9004)) [19]. Other scholars also explored and constructed many different combined models to improve the diagnostic accuracy of PCa [7,19–22].

It is well known that mpMRI is gradually spreading in the diagnostic application of PCa [23]. There are a lot of authors that have studied it and have offered interesting results in this regard. Grey et al. derived the negative predictive value of 97.7% for the PI-RADS score in the diagnosis of CSPCa [24]. They thought the PI-RADS scoring could be used in the decision-making process for detecting CSPCa. A systematic review from the Cochrane Database illustrated the benefit of detecting more CSPCa in mpMRI-targeted biopsies with a sensitivity of 0.80 (95% CI: 0.69–0.87) and a specificity of 0.94 (95% CI: 0.90–0.97) [25]. Mendhiratta et al. reported that targeted biopsy based on the mpMRI could detect more CSPCa than systematic biopsy (88.6% vs. 77.3%, p=0.037), which reflected the strong predictive efficiency of mpMRI in CSPCa [6]. The clinical application of mpMRI and the criteria for PI-RADS scoring are described in the ESUR prostate MR guidelines, providing clinicians with further improvements in the learning of mpMRI as well [26].

In this study, we developed clinical prediction models and devised nomograms using the combination of PHI, PI-RADS scores, and other important clinical predictors and developed a website that promotes our nomograms. For patients with elevated PSA but low predictive probability, measures such as active monitoring can be used.

Prostate biopsy is already a routine procedure and can be performed in many hospital outpatient operating rooms. With the widespread of transperineal prostate biopsy techniques, complications such as sepsis have decreased [27]. However, in some elderly patients with other diseases or poor coagulation function, prostate biopsy under local anesthesia still carries a high risk of bleeding. Therefore, a clinical predictive tool should be used to determine whether to perform active monitoring or to perform biopsy under close supervision.

Prior studies have constructed a number of nomograms that incorporate PHI and other clinical risk factors or PI-RADS and other clinical risk factors for PCa or CSPCa [20–22]. The superiority of the combined diagnosis of PHI and PI-RADS has also been demonstrated in several studies [19,28]. However, no studies constructed nomograms with the combination of PHI, PI-RADS scores, and other clinically significant predictive factors. Considering previous studies and the usefulness as well as the convenience of a clinical predictive model, we included four independent predictive factors in detecting PCa: age, PHI, PI-RADS, and PV. In predicting the positive rate of CSPCa, four predictive factors were included: age, PHI, PI-RADS, and Log PSAD. Although age had a P value of 0.084 for PCa in the univariable regression analysis, we still decided to include age in the model because age has been clinically identified as a risk factor in the development of PCa [29]. According to several observational studies, the diagnosis of patients with older age for PCa is associated with a poor prognosis [30,31]. As the (-2) proPSA was found in 1997, PHI is gradually becoming an effective means of screening for PCa [32] and has shown good AUC in detecting PCa and CSPCa [9,33]. As mentioned above, the nomogram studied in this study is more applicable to patients with TPSA between 4 and 20 ng/mL who are able to undergo the PHI test as well as the mpMRI examination. Although the applicability conditions are more stringent, it is beneficial to increase the detection rate of patients in this TPSA interval.

There are many previous nomograms for predicting PCa and studies combining PHI and PI-RADS score for detecting PCa [19,22]. Although the benefits of combining PHI with mpMRI are well recognized, the nomogram combining PHI with mpMRI has not been studied. As compared to previously published PCa and CSPCa predictive models, our study offers the following advantages. First, we visualized the prediction model as nomograms and developed a website with an operation interface for our nomogram on 20 August 2022, (https://zhouyonghengql.shinyapps.io/PCa_DynNom/), (https://zhouyonghengql.shinyapps.io/CSPCa_DynNomapp/), which greatly improved in terms of efficiency, accuracy, and clinical usability as a result of this optimization. Secondly, the combination of serum-specific biomarkers PHI and mpMRI also enables the combined diagnosis of physiological and anatomical functions, which can reduce the number of unnecessary biopsies by more than half.

It is worth mentioning that in our study, we analyzed the sensitivity and specificity of different cutoff values of PHI, and we found that as the cutoff value of PHI increased, the missed PCa and CSPCa also increased gradually. However, for the cut-off value of PHI of 35 [8], which is commonly used in clinical practice, our study found that its specificity is low, and it is necessary to appropriately increase the threshold of PHI for the detection of cancer. When the prediction rate for PCa by the nomogram is greater than 27%, our study suggests that prostate biopsy should be performed in this population with a low risk of missing CSPCa.

The following limitations were also included in our study. First, although this study is a prospective multicenter cohort study, the population sample size of our study was small, which may have some limitations. Secondly, there are many clinical studies that are still controversial and have not reached a consensus on the definition of CSPCa, and the GS $\geq$ 3 + 4 seems to be prevalent in most recent criteria [15,34]. We, therefore, used the definition in our study. In addition, maximum core length was used in the definition of CSPCa; however, we did not incorporate it into the final analysis, as it was not available for all patients. The use of a nomogram in this study can predict the probability of developing CSPCa before biopsy and can provide good treatment advice to patients. However, this study did not correlate the predictive results of the nomogram with the risk of CSPCa at the time of radical prostatectomy or the risk of adverse pathological features of radical prostatectomy, which remains a direction for future research and has considerable clinical implications. Finally, a larger sample and external validation are still needed to prove our conclusions and update our nomograms.

5. Conclusions

The combined diagnosis of PHI and PI-RADS can avoid more unnecessary biopsies. The nomogram with the combination of age, PHI, PV, and PI-RADS could improve the detection of PCa, and the nomogram with the combination of age, PHI, PI-RADS, and Log PSAD could improve the detection of CSPCa.

Supplementary Materials: The following supporting information can be downloaded at: https://www.mdpi.com/article/10.3390/jcm12010339/s1.

Author Contributions: Conceptualization, Y.Z. (Yongheng Zhou) and Y.Z. (Yaofeng Zhu); methodology, Q.F.; software, Z.S.; validation, K.Z., W.Q., and S.G.; formal analysis, W.W.; investigation, J.C.; resources, X.J.; data curation, R.L.; writing—original draft preparation, Y.Z. (Yongheng Zhou); writing—review and editing, S.C.; visualization, S.C; supervision, B.S.; project administration, B.S.; funding acquisition, Y.Z. (Yaofeng Zhu) and B.S. All authors have read and agreed to the published version of the manuscript.

Funding: This research was funded by the National Natural Science Foundation of China, grant numbers 81970661 and 82170790; the Natural Science Foundation of Shandong Province, grant number ZR2021MH318.

Institutional Review Board Statement: The study was conducted in accordance with the Declaration of Helsinki and approved by the Institutional Review Board of QILU Hospital of Shandong University (KYLL-202011-095-2 and April 12, 2021).

Informed Consent Statement: Informed consent was obtained from all subjects involved in the study.

Data Availability Statement: The datasets analyzed during the current study are available in the QILU Hospital of Shandong University.

Conflicts of Interest: The authors declare no conflict of interest.

References

1. Siegel, R.L.; Miller, K.D.; Fuchs, H.E.; Jemal, A. Cancer statistics, 2022. *CA A Cancer J. Clin.* **2022**, *72*, 7–33. [CrossRef] [PubMed]
2. Albertsen, P.C. Prostate cancer screening with prostate-specific antigen: Where are we going? *Cancer* **2018**, *124*, 453–455. [CrossRef]
3. Catalona, W.J.; Partin, A.W.; Sanda, M.G.; Wei, J.T.; Klee, G.G.; Bangma, C.H.; Slawin, K.M.; Marks, L.S.; Loeb, S.; Broyles, D.L.; et al. A Multicenter Study of [-2]Pro-Prostate Specific Antigen Combined With Prostate Specific Antigen and Free Prostate Specific Antigen for Prostate Cancer Detection in the 2.0 to 10.0 ng/mL Prostate Specific Antigen Range. *J. Urol.* **2011**, *185*, 1650–1655. [CrossRef] [PubMed]
4. Vickers, A.J.; Vertosick, E.A.; Sjoberg, D.D. Value of a Statistical Model Based on Four Kallikrein Markers in Blood, Commercially Available as 4Kscore, in All Reasonable Prostate Biopsy Subgroups. *Eur. Urol.* **2018**, *74*, 535–536. [CrossRef] [PubMed]

5. Tan, G.H.; Nason, G.; Ajib, K.; Woon, D.T.S.; Herrera-Caceres, J.; Alhunaidi, O.; Perlis, N. Smarter screening for prostate cancer. *World J. Urol.* **2019**, *37*, 991–999. [CrossRef] [PubMed]
6. Mendhiratta, N.; Rosenkrantz, A.B.; Meng, X.; Wysock, J.S.; Fenstermaker, M.; Huang, R.; Deng, F.M.; Melamed, J.; Zhou, M.; Huang, W.C.; et al. Magnetic Resonance Imag-ing-Ultrasound Fusion Targeted Prostate Biopsy in a Consecutive Cohort of Men with No Previous Biopsy: Reduction of Over Detection through Improved Risk Stratification. *J. Urol.* **2015**, *194*, 1601–1606. [CrossRef] [PubMed]
7. Zhou, Y.; Qi, W.; Cui, J.; Zhong, M.; Lv, G.; Qu, S.; Chen, S.; Li, R.; Shi, B.; Zhu, Y. Construction and Comparison of Different Models in Detecting Prostate Cancer and Clinically Significant Prostate Cancer. *Front. Oncol.* **2022**, *12*, 911725. [CrossRef]
8. Chiu, P.K.-F.; Ng, C.-F.; Semjonow, A.; Zhu, Y.; Vincendeau, S.; Houlgatte, A.; Lazzeri, M.; Guazzoni, G.; Stephan, C.; Haese, A.; et al. A Multicentre Evaluation of the Role of the Prostate Health Index (PHI) in Regions with Differing Prevalence of Prostate Cancer: Adjustment of PHI Reference Ranges is Needed for European and Asian Settings. *Eur. Urol.* **2019**, *75*, 558–561. [CrossRef]
9. Mikolajczyk, S.D.; Grauer, L.S.; Millar, L.S.; Hill, T.M.; Kumar, A.; Rittenhouse, H.G.; Wolfert, R.L.; Saedi, M.S. A precursor form of PSA (pPSA) is a com-ponent of the free PSA in prostate cancer serum. *Urology* **1997**, *50*, 710–714. [CrossRef]
10. Turkbey, B.; Rosenkrantz, A.B.; Haider, M.A.; Padhani, A.R.; Villeirs, G.; Macura, K.J.; Tempany, C.M.; Choyke, P.L.; Cornud, F.; Margolis, D.J.; et al. Prostate Imaging Reporting and Data System Version 2.1: 2019 Update of Prostate Imaging Reporting and Data System Version 2. *Eur. Urol.* **2019**, *76*, 340–351. [CrossRef]
11. Nilsson, O.; Peter, A.T.; Andersson, I.; Nilsson, K.; Grundström, B.; Karlsson, B. Antigenic determinants of prostate-specific antigen (PSA) and development of assays specific for different forms of PSA. *Br. J. Cancer* **1997**, *75*, 789–797. [CrossRef]
12. Weinreb, J.C.; Barentsz, J.O.; Choyke, P.L.; Cornud, F.; Haider, M.A.; Macura, K.J.; Margolis, D.; Schnall, M.D.; Shtern, F.; Tempany, C.M.; et al. PI-RADS Prostate Imaging—Reporting and Data System: 2015, Version 2. *Eur. Urol.* **2016**, *69*, 16–40. [CrossRef] [PubMed]
13. Padhani, A.R.; Weinreb, J.; Rosenkrantz, A.B.; Villeirs, G.; Turkbey, B.; Barentsz, J. Prostate Imaging-Reporting and Data System Steering Committee: PI-RADS v2 Status Update and Future Directions. *Eur. Urol.* **2019**, *75*, 385–396. [CrossRef]
14. Epstein, J.I.; Egevad, L.; Amin, M.B.; Delahunt, B.; Srigley, J.R.; Humphrey, P.A. The 2014 International Society of Urological Pathology (ISUP) Consensus Conference on Gleason Grading of Prostatic Carcinoma: Definition of Grading Patterns and Proposal for a New Grading System. *Am. J. Surg. Pathol.* **2016**, *40*, 244–252. [CrossRef]
15. Matoso, A.; Epstein, J. Defining clinically significant prostate cancer on the basis of pathological findings. *Histopathology* **2019**, *74*, 135–145. [CrossRef]
16. Obuchowski, N.A.; Bullen, J.A. Receiver operating characteristic (ROC) curves: Review of methods with applications in diagnostic medicine. *Phys. Med. Biol.* **2018**, *63*, 07TR01. [CrossRef] [PubMed]
17. Rosenfeld, J.P.; Donchin, E. Resampling (bootstrapping) the mean: A definite do. *Psychophysiology* **2015**, *52*, 969–972. [CrossRef] [PubMed]
18. Noureldin, M.; Eldred-Evans, D.; Khoo, C.C.; Winkler, M.; Sokhi, H.; Tam, H.; Ahmed, H.U. Review article: MRI-targeted biopsies for prostate cancer diagnosis and management. *World J. Urol.* **2021**, *39*, 57–63. [CrossRef]
19. Hsieh, P.-F.; Li, W.-J.; Lin, W.-C.; Chang, H.; Chang, C.-H.; Huang, C.-P.; Yang, C.-R.; Chen, W.-C.; Chang, Y.-H.; Wu, H.-C. Combining prostate health index and multiparametric magnetic resonance imaging in the diagnosis of clinically significant prostate cancer in an Asian population. *World J. Urol.* **2020**, *38*, 1207–1214. [CrossRef]
20. Foj, L.; Filella, X. Development and internal validation of a novel PHI-nomogram to identify aggressive prostate cancer. *Clin. Chim. Acta* **2020**, *501*, 174–178. [CrossRef]
21. Sun, J.; Zhang, Z.; OuYang, J. A novel nomogram combined PIRADS v2 and neutrophil-to-lymphocyte ratio to predict the risk of clinically significant prostate cancer in men with PSA < 10 ng/mL at first biopsy. *Urol. Oncol. Semin. Orig. Investig.* **2020**, *38*, 401–409. [CrossRef]
22. Zhou, Z.H.; Liu, F.; Wang, W.J.; Liu, X.; Sun, L.J.; Zhu, Y.; Ye, D.W.; Zhang, G.M. Development and validation of a nomogram including lympho-cyte-to-monocyte ratio for initial prostate biopsy: A double-center retrospective study. *Asian J. Androl.* **2021**, *23*, 41–46.
23. van der Leest, M.; Cornel, E.; Israël, B.; Hendriks, R.; Padhani, A.R.; Hoogenboom, M.; Zamecnik, P.; Bakker, D.; Setiasti, A.Y.; Veltman, J.; et al. Head-to-head Comparison of Transrectal Ultrasound-guided Prostate Biopsy Versus Multiparametric Prostate Resonance Imaging with Subsequent Magnetic Reso-nance-guided Biopsy in Biopsy-naïve Men with Elevated Prostate-specific Antigen: A Large Prospective Multicenter Clinical Study. *Eur. Urol.* **2019**, *75*, 570–578. [PubMed]
24. Grey, A.D.; Chana, M.S.; Popert, R.; Wolfe, K.; Liyanage, S.H.; Acher, P.L. Diagnostic accuracy of magnetic resonance imaging (MRI) prostate imaging reporting and data system (PI-RADS) scoring in a transperineal prostate biopsy setting. *Br. J. Urol.* **2015**, *115*, 728–735. [CrossRef] [PubMed]
25. Drost, F.-J.H.; Osses, D.F.; Nieboer, D.; Steyerberg, E.W.; Bangma, C.H.; Roobol, M.J.; Schoots, I.G. Prostate MRI, with or without MRI-targeted biopsy, and systematic biopsy for detecting prostate cancer. *Cochrane Database Syst. Rev.* **2019**, *4*, CD012663. [CrossRef] [PubMed]
26. Barentsz, J.O.; Richenberg, J.; Clements, R.; Choyke, P.; Verma, S.; Villeirs, G.; Rouviere, O.; Logager, V.; Fütterer, J.J. ESUR prostate MR guidelines 2012. *Eur. Radiol.* **2012**, *22*, 746–757. [CrossRef] [PubMed]

27. Berry, B.; Parry, M.G.; Sujenthiran, A.; Nossiter, J.; Cowling, T.E.; Aggarwal, A.; Cathcart, P.; Payne, H.; van der Meulen, J.; Clarke, N.; et al. Comparison of complications after transrectal and transperineal prostate biopsy: A national population-based study. *BJU Int.* **2020**, *126*, 97–103. [CrossRef]
28. Schwen, Z.R.; Mamawala, M.; Tosoian, J.J.; Druskin, S.C.; Ross, A.E.; Sokoll, L.J.; Epstein, J.I.; Carter, H.B.; Gorin, M.A.; Pavlovich, C.P. Prostate Health Index and multiparametric magnetic resonance imaging to predict prostate cancer grade reclassification in active surveillance. *BJU Int.* **2020**, *126*, 373–378. [CrossRef]
29. Mottet, N.; van den Bergh, R.C.; Briers, E.; Van den Broeck, T.; Cumberbatch, M.G.; De Santis, M.; Fanti, S.; Fossati, N.; Gandaglia, G.; Gillessen, S.; et al. EAU-EANM-ESTRO-ESUR-SIOG Guidelines on Prostate Cancer-2020 Update. Part 1: Screening, Diagnosis, and Local Treatment with Curative Intent. *Eur. Urol.* **2021**, *79*, 243–262. [CrossRef]
30. Abdollah, F.; Sun, M.; Thuret, R.; Jeldres, C.; Tian, Z.; Briganti, A.; Shariat, S.F.; Perrotte, P.; Rigatti, P.; Montorsi, F.; et al. A Competing-Risks Analysis of Survival After Alternative Treatment Modalities for Prostate Cancer Patients: 1988–2006. *Eur. Urol.* **2011**, *59*, 88–95. [CrossRef]
31. Bechis, S.K.; Carroll, P.R.; Cooperberg, M.R. Impact of age at diagnosis on prostate cancer treatment and survival. *J. Clin. Oncol. Off. J. Am. Soc. Clin. Oncol.* **2011**, *29*, 235–241. [CrossRef] [PubMed]
32. Barisiene, M.; Bakavicius, A.; Stanciute, D.; Jurkeviciene, J.; Zelvys, A.; Ulys, A.; Vitkus, D.; Jankevicius, F. Prostate Health Index and Prostate Health Index Density as Diagnostic Tools for Improved Prostate Cancer Detection. *BioMed Res. Int.* **2020**, *2020*, 9872146. [CrossRef] [PubMed]
33. Loeb, S.; Sanda, M.G.; Broyles, D.L.; Shin, S.S.; Bangma, C.H.; Wei, J.T.; Partin, A.W.; Klee, G.G.; Slawin, K.M.; Marks, L.S.; et al. The Prostate Health Index Selectively Identifies Clinically Significant Prostate Cancer. *J. Urol.* **2015**, *193*, 1163–1169. [CrossRef] [PubMed]
34. Fütterer, J.J.; Briganti, A.; De Visschere, P.; Emberton, M.; Giannarini, G.; Kirkham, A.; Taneja, S.S.; Thoeny, H.; Villeirs, G.; Villers, A. Can Clinically Significant Prostate Cancer Be Detected with Multiparametric Magnetic Resonance Imaging? A Systematic Review of the Literature. *Eur. Urol.* **2015**, *68*, 1045–1053. [CrossRef]

Journal of
Clinical Medicine

MDPI

Article

Diagnostic Efficiency of Pan-Immune-Inflammation Value to Predict Prostate Cancer in Patients with Prostate-Specific Antigen between 4 and 20 ng/mL

Meikai Zhu [1,†], Yongheng Zhou [1,†], Zhifeng Liu [2], Zhiwen Jiang [1], Wenqiang Qi [1], Shouzhen Chen [1], Wenfu Wang [1], Benkang Shi [1] and Yaofeng Zhu [1,*]

[1] Department of Urology, Qilu Hospital of Shandong University, Jinan 250012, China
[2] Department of Urology, Tai'an City Central Hospital, Tai'an 271000, China
* Correspondence: feng2209@email.sdu.edu.cn
† These authors contributed equally to this work and share first authorship.

Abstract: Introduction: To evaluate the predictive value of the pan-immune-inflammation value (PIV) and other systemic inflammatory markers, including the neutrophil-to-lymphocyte ratio (NLR), derived neutrophil-to-lymphocyte ratio (dNLR), monocyte-to-lymphocyte ratio (MLR), platelet-to-lymphocyte ratio (PLR), and systemic immune-inflammation index (SII), for prostate cancer (PCa) and clinically significant prostate cancer (CSPCa) in patients with a prostate-specific antigen (PSA) value between 4 and 20 ng/mL. Patients and Methods: The clinical data of 319 eligible patients who underwent prostate biopsies in our hospital from August 2019 to June 2022 were retrospectively analyzed. CSPCa was defined as a "Gleason grade group of $\geq$2". A univariable logistic regression analysis and multivariable logistic regression analysis were conducted to analyze the association between the PIV, SII, MLR, and PCa/CSPCa. For the inflammatory indicators included in the multivariable logistic regression analysis, we constructed models by combining the separate inflammatory indicator and other significant predictors and compared the area under the curve (AUC). A nomogram based on the PIV for PCa was developed. Results: We included 148 PCa patients (including 127 CSPCa patients) and 171 non-PCa patients in total. The patients with PCa were older, had higher MLR, SII, PIV, and total PSA (TPSA) values, consumed more alcohol, and had lower free/total PSA (f/T) values than the other patients. Compared with the non-CSPCa group, the CSPCa group had higher BMI, MLR, PIV, TPSA values, consumed more alcohol, and had lower f/T values. The univariable regression analysis showed that drinking history, higher MLR, PIV, and TPSA values, and lower f/T values were independent predictors of PCa and CSPCa. The AUC of the PIV in the multivariable logistic regression model was higher than those of the MLR and SII. In addition, the diagnostic value of the PIV + PSA for PCa was better than the PSA value. However, the diagnostic value for CSPCa was not significantly different from that of using PSA alone, while the AUC of the PIV + PSA was higher than the individual indicator of the PSA value. Conclusions: Our study suggests that for the patients who were diagnosed with PSA values between 4 and 20 ng/mL, the PIV and MLR are potential indicators for predicting PCa and CSPCa. In addition, our study indicates that the new inflammatory index PIV has clinical value in the diagnosis of PCa and CSPCa.

Keywords: PIV; systemic inflammatory markers; prostate biopsy; diagnosis; prostate cancer

1. Introduction

Prostate cancer (PCa) is a common malignant tumor worldwide and is the second cause of cancer-related death in men [1]. Prostate-specific antigen (PSA) is a major biomarker for PCa diagnosis. Currently, PCa is usually determined by systematic ultrasound-guided biopsies prompted by elevated levels of PSA in serum [2]. However, only 25% of men with elevated PSA levels are diagnosed with PCa because of the poor specificity of PSA, which means that 75% of patients undergo unnecessary and potentially harmful follow-up tests, such as biopsies, especially for men with PSA values between 4.0 and 20.0 ng/mL (low and medium clinical risk category) [3]. In order to make up for this defect, many biomarkers of PCa have been developed successively, such as the prostate health index, 4K score, SelectMDx, and ExoDx Prostate IntelliScoreTM [4]. However, these experimental methods have some disadvantages, such as high costs, which means they cannot be routinely used for the detection of PCa [5].

In recent years, it has become increasingly accepted that certain systemic inflammatory reactions may play a significant role in tumor promotion and progression. Tumor-related systemic inflammatory markers, including the neutrophil-to-lymphocyte ratio (NLR), derived neutrophil-to-lymphocyte ratio (dNLR), monocyte-to-lymphocyte ratio (MLR), platelet-to-lymphocyte ratio (PLR), and systemic immune-inflammation index (SII), have gained attention as diagnostic tools for tumors [6,7].

The pan-immune-inflammation value (PIV), a novel equation that includes the neutrophil count, platelet count, monocyte count, and lymphocyte count from peripheral blood, has been reported as a potential prognostic biomarker in several cancers [8]. There have been no studies of the diagnostic value of the PIV in PCa.

In the present study, our primary goal was to investigate whether the PIV could be used to predict PCa in patients with PSA levels between 4.0 and 20.0 ng/mL. We also verified the diagnostic efficacy of the NLR, dNLR, MLR, PLR and SII in PCa.

2. Materials and Methods

2.1. Patient Selection Information Collection

This is a retrospective study that was approved by the Institutional Ethics Review Board of QILU Hospital of Shandong University (KYLL-202111-107). We obtained the information of all patients who received prostate biopsies with PSA levels of 4.0–20.0 ng/mL in our hospital from August 2019 to June 2022 from the electronic medical record system at our hospital. All patients underwent routine blood tests with serum PSA derivative (including total PSA [TPSA] and free PSA [fPSA]) within 2 weeks before their biopsies. Patients with one or more of the following conditions were excluded from this study: (I) Patients with other malignancies, known infections, and hematological diseases; (II) Patients who had had prostate surgery (such as transurethral resection of the prostate) before their biopsies; (III) Patients with pathological diagnoses of atypical small acinar proliferation and prostatic intraepithelial neoplasia; and (IV) Patients with incomplete clinical data. Then, we collected the following data of eligible patients from the medical records: age, body mass index (BMI), history of tobacco and alcohol use, medical history, blood test results with serum PSA, histopathologic findings, and Gleason score.

2.2. Biopsy Method and Pathological Examination

All patients had received prostate mpMRI before biopsies, which were performed by two uroradiologists with a minimum of three years of experience using a 3.0 T scanner. Experienced members of the surgical team retrospectively performed imaging assessments to reach a consensus on the imaging findings to determine the biopsy methods. Finally, all patients underwent transrectal biopsies or transperineal biopsies under local anesthesia. The prostate biopsies were performed with 12 + 3 cores (on the basis of 12 systematic cores, with the remaining core at the suspicious area shown on the MRI by cognitive fusion biopsies). Then, pathological tissues from the biopsy specimens were analyzed by two experienced uropathologists according to International Society of Urological Pathology consensus guidelines within one week post-surgery.

2.3. Data Management

The patients were classified into non-PCa group and PCa group based on the histopathologic results. In addition, we divided the patients into CSPCa group and non-CSPCa group. The definition of clinically significant prostate cancer (CSPCa) was "Gleason grade group of ≥2" [9]. The PIV, NLR, dNLR, MLR, PLR and SII were defined as "neutrophil count × platelet count × monocyte count/lymphocyte count", "neutrophil count/lymphocyte count", "neutrophil count/(leukocyte count–neutrophil count)", "monocyte count/lymphocyte count", "platelet count/lymphocyte count" and "neutrophil count × platelet count/lymphocyte count", respectively. All the above blood cell counts were obtained within two weeks before biopsies.

2.4. Statistical Analysis

All continuous variables were tested for normality. The continuous variables that met the normality test used the Student's *t*-test and the variables with skewed distribution used the Mann–Whitney *U*-test. Continuous variables with normal distribution were reported with mean ± SD and continuous variables with skewed distribution were reported as median (IQR). Categorical variables were analyzed using Chi-square tests and reported as numbers (percentages). Univariable and multivariable logistic regression analyses were conducted to identify the independently predictive factors for PCa and CSPCa. The predictors with p values less than 0.05 in univariable logistic regression were included in multivariable logistic regression. We constructed different models using different inflammatory factors and other clinical variables and compared the performance of different models. A p value less than 0.05 was considered statistically significant. We developed a PCa risk nomogram, including PIV for prostate biopsy. The calibration was examined by the calibration curves. Decision curve analysis (DCA) was performed to assess the clinical usefulness of the nomogram by calculating the net benefits. The DeLong test was used to compare the differences in AUC. SPSS V.25.0 (IBM Corp, Armonk, NY, USA) and R statistical software (Version 4.1.0) were used to perform statistical analysis.

3. Results

3.1. Clinical Demographics of the Eligible Patients

A total of 319 individual patients met the study's entry criteria and were included in the study. The mean age, PIV, TPSA levels were 66 years, 197.04, and 9.23ng/mL, respectively. PCa was detected in 148 patients (including 127 patients with CSPCa). The characteristics and laboratory values of the patients are shown in Table 1.

Table 1. Characteristic baseline.

Variable	Overall (n = 319)	Non-PCa (n = 171)	PCa (n = 148)	p Value	Non-CSPCa (n = 192)	CSPCa (n = 127)	p Value
Age, year	66.00 (61.00–72.00)	65.00 (59.00–71.00)	67.00 (62.00–73.00)	0.011	66 (60–72)	66 (62–73)	0.285
BMI, kg/m^2	24.80 (22.99–26.57)	24.57 (22.78–26.12)	25.02 (23.54–27.03)	0.064	24.57 (22.78–26.12)	25.10 (23.56–27.06)	0.025
SH (%)				0.191			0.189
Y	90 (28.2)	43 (25.1)	47 (31.8)		49 (25.5)	41 (32.3)	
N	229 (71.8)	128 (74.9)	101 (68.2)		143 (74.5)	86 (67.7)	
AH (%)				0.015			0.016
Y	87 (27.3)	37 (21.6)	50 (33.8)		43 (22.4)	44 (34.6)	
N	232 (72.7)	134 (78.4)	98 (66.2)		149 (77.6)	83 (65.4)	
NLR	1.90 (1.52–2.48)	1.88 (1.44–2.58)	1.93 (1.59–2.47)	0.171	1.89 (1.44–2.51)	1.93 (1.58–2.48)	0.244
dNLR	1.37 (1.10–1.76)	1.40 (1.09–1.86)	1.36 (1.12–1.72)	0.679	1.40 (1.09–1.78)	1.35 (1.11–1.73)	0.720
MLR	0.27 (0.22–0.34)	0.25 (0.20–0.30)	0.30 (0.23–0.39)	<0.001	0.26 (0.20–0.31)	0.30 (0.23–0.39)	<0.001
PLR	122.98 (98.58–150.50)	120 (96.11–143.86)	132.30 (101.16–153.20)	0.053	121.10 (96.34–144.56)	132.54 (100.00–153.21)	0.099
SII, 10^9	411.79 (316.84–531.05)	393.89 (293.30–501.92)	427.26 (339.28–544.45)	0.030	402.14 (305.01–521.53)	423.77 (328.05–531.39)	0.145
PIV, 10^{18}	197.04 (134.56–289.76)	171.54 (123.48–244.10)	229.62 (152.47–329.29)	<0.001	181.04 (125.45–251.83)	228.49 (151.17–325.61)	0.001
Hb, g/L	147 (138–154)	148 (139–155)	147 (137–154)	0.448	148 (139–155)	147 (137–154)	0.484

Table 1. *Cont.*

Variable	Overall (n = 319)	Non-PCa (n = 171)	PCa (n = 148)	p Value	Non-CSPCa (n = 192)	CSPCa (n = 127)	p Value
TPSA, ng/mL	9.23 (6.71–12.53)	8.40 (6.07–10.93)	10.76 (7.65–14.27)	<0.001	8.40 (6.10–11.07)	11.05 (8.01–14.52)	<0.001
fPSA, ng/mL	1.20 (0.82–1.74)	1.22 (0.86–1.76)	1.14 (0.79–1.66)	0.792	1.23 (0.85–1.78)	1.14 (0.80–1.60)	0.609
f/T	0.14 (0.10–0.18)	0.15 (0.11–0.19)	0.12 (0.79–1.66)	<0.001	0.15 (0.11–0.19)	0.11 (0.09–0.16)	<0.001

BMI: body mass index; SH: smoking history; AH: alcohol history; NLR: neutrophil-to-lymphocyte ratio; dNLR: derived neutrophil-to-lymphocyte ratio; MLR: monocyte-to-lymphocyte ratio; PLR: platelet-to-lymphocyte ratio; SII: systemic immune-inflammation index; PIV: pan-immune-inflammation value; HB: hemoglobin; TPSA: total prostatic specific antigen; fPSA: free prostatic specific antigen; f/T: free/ total prostatic specific antigen ratio; PCa: prostate cancer; CSPCa: clinically significant prostate cancer, which was defined as Gleason grade ≥ 2.

The mean age (67.00 vs 65.00, $p = 0.011$), MLR (0.30 vs 0.25, $p < 0.001$), SII (427.26 vs 393.89, $p = 0.03$), PIV (229.62 vs 171.54, $p < 0.001$), and TPSA (10.76 vs 8.40, $p < 0.001$) of the PCa group were significantly higher than those of the non-PCa group. In addition, the proportion of patients with a history of alcohol use in the PCa group was also higher than that in the non-PCa group (Table 1).

The CSPCa group had higher BMI, MLR, PIV and TPSA levels than the non-CSPCa group. However, there was no significant difference in the age or SII between the two groups. Moreover, there was no statistically significant difference in the NLR, dNLR, and PLR between the PCa group vs non-PCa group as well as the CSPCa group vs non-CSPCa group (Table 1).

3.2. Univariable and Multivariable Analyses of Clinical Indicators

We conducted univariable and multivariable logistic regression analyses to determine the predictive factors of the clinical indicators. Age, history of alcohol use, MLR, SII, PIV, TPSA and f/T values were significant predictors of PCa according to the results of the univariable regression analysis (Table 2). Then we chose all the significant variables in the univariable regression analysis and subjected them to the multivariable regression analysis. The results showed that history of alcohol use, higher age, higher MLR and TPSA values, and lower f/T values had a greater probability for the detection of PCa (Table 2).

Table 2. Univariable and multivariable analyses of clinical indicators.

PCa	Univariable Regression Analysis		Multivariable Regression Analysis		CSPCa	Univariable Regression Analysis		Multivariable Regression Analysis	
	OR (95% CI)	p Value	OR (95% CI)	p Value		OR (95% CI)	p Value	OR (95% CI)	p Value
Age	1.035 (1.008–1.064)	0.012	1.046 (1.014–1.079)	0.005	Age	1.015 (0.988–1.042)	0.284		
BMI	1.075 (0.995–1.160)	0.066			BMI	1.090 (1.007–1.179)	0.032	1.114 (1.021–1.217)	0.016
SH					SH				
Y	1.385 (0.849–2.259)	0.192			Y	1.391 (0.849–2.279)	0.190		
N	1				N	1			
AH					AH				
Y	1.848 (1.122–3.042)	0.016	1.975 (1.141–3.416)	0.015	Y	1.837 (1.116–3.025)	0.017	1.706 (0.989–2.940)	0.055
N	1		1		N	1		1	
NLR	1.234 (0.936–1.629)	0.136			NLR	1.192 (0.903–1.574)	0.216		
dNLR	0.849 (0.636–1.134)	0.268			dNLR	0.862 (0.642–1.158)	0.324		
MLR	52.028 (7.377–366.922)	<0.001	16.513 (1.091–249.847)	0.043	MLR	27.469 (4.298–175.552)	<0.001	19.473 (1.557–243.616)	0.021
PLR	1.003 (0.998–1.008)	0.188			PLR	1.003 (0.998–1.007)	0.299		
SII	1.001 (1.000–1.002)	0.028	1.000 (0.998–1.002)	0.731	SII	1.001 (1.000–1.002)	0.053		

Table 2. *Cont.*

PCa	Univariable Regression Analysis		Multivariable Regression Analysis		CSPCa	Univariable Regression Analysis		Multivariable Regression Analysis	
	OR (95% CI)	p Value	OR (95% CI)	p Value		OR (95% CI)	p Value	OR (95% CI)	p Value
PIV	1.003 (1.001–1.004)	0.001	1.002 (0.998–1.005)	0.324	PIV	1.002 (1.001–1.003)	0.002	1.001 (0.999–1.003)	0.406
Hb	0.997 (0.983–1.011)	0.684			Hb	0.998 (0.984–1.013)	0.814		
TPSA	1.163 (1.094–1.236)	<0.001	1.138 (1.063–1.217)	<0.001	TPSA	1.158 (1.090–1.231)	<0.001	1.140 (1.067–1.218)	<0.001
fPSA	1.076 (0.794–1.459)	0.635			fPSA	0.941 (0.689–1.286)	0.704		
f/T	0.003 (0.000–0.096)	0.001	0.006 (0.000–0.413)	0.018	f/T	0.001 (0.000–0.028)	<0.001	0.004 (0.000–0.278)	0.010

BMI: body mass index; SH: smoking history; AH: alcohol history; NLR: neutrophil-to-lymphocyte ratio; dNLR: derived neutrophil-to-lymphocyte ratio; MLR: monocyte-to-lymphocyte ratio; PLR: platelet-to-lymphocyte ratio; SII: systemic immune-inflammation index; PIV: pan-immune-inflammation value; HB: hemoglobin; TPSA: total prostatic specific antigen; fPSA: free prostatic specific antigen; f/T: free/total prostatic specific antigen ratio; PCa: prostate cancer; CSPCa: clinically significant prostate cancer, which was defined as Gleason grade $\geq$ 2; OR: odds ratio; CI: CI: confidence interval.

In the univariable regression analysis between the CSPCa group and non-CSPCa group, we found that patients with higher BMIs, a greater history of alcohol use, higher MLR, PIV, and TPSA values, and lower f/T values were more likely to be diagnosed with CSPCa (Table 2). The independent variables with $p < 0.05$ in the univariable analysis were selected for the multivariable regression analysis. According to the result of the multivariable logistic regression analysis, higher BMI, MLR, and TPSA values and lower f/T values were the independent predictors of CSPCa (Table 2).

3.3. Multivariable Logistic Regression Analysis of Different Models of Inflammatory Markers

As mentioned above, we found that age, BMI, history of alchohol use, TPSA, f/T values were independent predictors of PCa or CSPCa. Therefore, we performed multivariable logistic regression analyses with MLR, SII, PIV, and other risk factors and constructed different models (Model A, Model B, Model C) (Table 3), respectively, to predict the outcomes of the biopsies. The AUC values (Figure 1) from high to low were Model C (AUC = 0.754, 95% CI: 0.701–0.808, p = 0.001), Model A (AUC = 0.750, 95% CI: 0.701–0.808, p < 0.001), and Model B (AUC = 0.745, 95% CI: 0.701–0.808, p = 0.008). This meant that among the three models, Model C had the highest diagnostic value for the detection of PCa, although the difference between them is not obvious. The specificity and sensitivity of Model C for the PCa values were 0.703 and 0.719 (Table 4), respectively. Similar results appeared in the group of CSPCa patients, which showed that Model C (AUC = 0.751, 95% CI: 0.696–0.806, p = 0.003) had the highest diagnostic value followed by Model A (AUC = 0.750, 95% CI: 0.696–0.804, p = 0.001) and Model B (AUC = 0.742, 95% CI: 0.686–0.798, p = 0.021) with a sensitivity and specificity of 0.669 and 0.750 (Table 4).

Table 3. Multivariable logistic regression analysis of different models of inflammatory markers.

PCa	Model A		Model B		Model C	
	OR (95% CI)	*p* Value	OR (95% CI)	*p* Value	OR (95% CI)	*p* Value
Age	1.048 (1.016–1.081)	0.003	1.056 (1.023–1.089)	0.001	1.055 (1.023–1.089)	0.001
BMI	1.106 (1.014–1.207)	0.023	1.111 (1.019–1.212)	0.017	1.110 (1.017–1.211)	0.019
AH		0.031		0.029		0.032
Y	1.841 (1.059–3.200)		1.841 (1.063–3.188)		1.832 (1.054–3.186)	
N	1		1		1	
MLR	59.057 (7.385–472.306)	<0.001	/		/	
SII	/		1.001 (1.000–1.003)	0.008	/	
PIV	/		/		1.003 (1.001–1.004)	0.001
TPSA	1.143 (1.068–1.223)	<0.001	1.138 (1.064–1.217)	<0.001	1.134 (1.061–1.213)	<0.001
f/T	0.004 (0.000–0.260)	0.009	0.003 (0.000–0.215)	0.007	0.004 (0.000–0.238)	0.008
AUC (95% CI)	0.750 (0.697–0.804)		0.745 (0.701–0.808)		0.754 (0.701–0.808)	
CSPCa						
Age	1.025 (0.994–1.053)	0.111	1.033 (1.002–1.065)	0.040	1.032 (1.001–1.064)	0.045
BMI	1.119 (1.024–1.222)	0.013	1.123 (1.028–1.226)	0.010	1.122 (1.027–1.226)	0.011
AH		0.049		0.050		0.055
Y	1.732 (1.002–2.996)		1.721 (1.000–1.226)		1.706 (0.988–2.945)	
N	1		1		1	
MLR	34.010 (4.624–250.170)	0.001	/		/	
SII	/		1.001 (1.000–1.002)	0.021	/	
PIV	/		/		1.002 (1.001–1.004)	0.003
TPSA	1.135 (1.062–1.213)	<0.001	1.131 (1.059–1.208)	<0.001	1.126 (1.054–1.203)	<0.001
f/T	0.002 (0.000–0.122)	0.004	0.001 (0.000–0.100)	0.003	0.001 (0.000–0.104)	0.003
AUC (95% CI)	0.750 (0.696–0.804)		0.742 (0.686–0.798)		0.751 (0.696–0.806)	

AH: alcohol history; MLR: monocyte-to-lymphocyte ratio; SII: systemic immune-inflammation index; PIV: pan-immune-inflammation value; TPSA: total prostatic specific antigen; f/T: free/total prostatic specific antigen ratio; AUC: the area under curve; CI: Confidence interval; OR: odds ratio; PCa: prostate cancer; CSPCa: clinically significant prostate cancer, which was defined as Gleason grade ≥ 2.

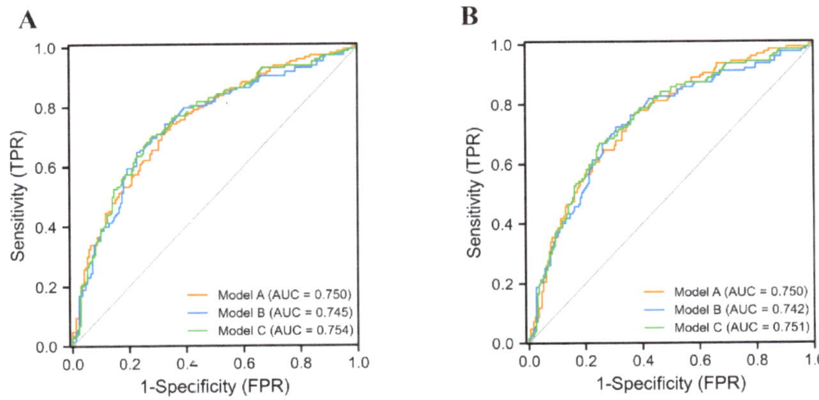

Figure 1. The AUC curves of different models based on SII, MLR, and PIV, respectively, in prostate cancer (**A**) and clinically significant prostate cancer (**B**).

Table 4. ROC curve analysis of variables.

Variables	AUC (95% CI)	Cut-Off	Sensitivity	Specificity	PPV	NPV	Youden Index
PCa							
MLR	0.636 (0.576–0.697)	0.302	0.493	0.754	0.635	0.632	0.248
SII	0.570 (0.508–0.633)	374.674	0.703	0.444	0.523	0.633	0.147
PIV	0.639 (0.578–0.700)	219.616	0.547	0.708	0.618	0.644	0.255
TPSA	0.657 (0.596–0.717)	11.577	0.453	0.819	0.684	0.633	0.271
Model A	0.750 (0.697–0.804)	0.382	0.709	0.684	0.660	0.731	0.394
Model B	0.745 (0.690–0.800)	0.425	0.649	0.772	0.711	0.717	0.421
Model C	0.754 (0.701–0.808)	0.402	0.703	0.719	0.684	0.737	0.422
CSPCa							
MLR	0.625 (0.563–0.688)	0.302	0.504	0.734	0.557	0.691	0.238
SII	0.548 (0.484–0.612)	365.367	0.717	0.401	0.442	0.681	0.118
PIV	0.615 (0.552–0.678)	210.291	0.567	0.656	0.522	0.696	0.223
TPSA	0.661 (0.599–0.724)	11.577	0.480	0.807	0.622	0.701	0.288
Model A	0.750 (0.696–0.804)	0.362	0.772	0.625	0.576	0.805	0.397
Model B	0.742 (0.685–0.798)	0.399	0.724	0.693	0.609	0.792	0.417
Model C	0.751 (0.696–0.806)	0.428	0.669	0.750	0.639	0.774	0.419

MLR: monocyte-to-lymphocyte ratio; SII: systemic immune-inflammation index; PIV: pan-immune-inflammation value; AUC: the area under curve; ROC: receiver operating characteristic; PCa: prostate cancer; CSPCa: clinically significant prostate cancer, which was defined as Gleason grade $\geq$ 2; PPV: positive predictive value; NPV: negative predictive value; Model A: multivariable logistic regression analysis based on the MLR; Model B: multivariable logistic regression analysis based on the SII; Model C: multivariable logistic regression analysis based on the PIV.

3.4. ROC Curve Analysis of Variables

In order to evaluate the diagnostic value of a single variable for PCa and CSPCa, we performed the ROC-AUC analysis of the MLR, SII, PIV and TPSA. The detailed results of the analysis are presented in Table 4, Figures 2 and 3. TPSA (AUC = 0.657, 95% CI: 0.596–0.717) had the highest predictive value for PCa values according to the parameters of the analysis. The AUC values for the MLR, SII, and PIV were 0.636 (95% CI: 0.576–0.697), 0.570 (95% CI: 0.508–0.633), and 0.639 (95% CI: 0.578–0.700), respectively. In the group of CSPCa, the ROC curve analysis showed that the AUCs of MLR, SII, PIV, and TPSA were 0.625 (95% CI: 0.563–0.688), 0.548 (95% CI: 0.484–0.612), 0.615 (95% CI: 0.552–0.678), and 0.661 (95% CI: 0.599–0.724), respectively. In summary, TPSA has the highest diagnostic value for both PCA and CSPCa. At the same time, the PIV and MLR are also the powerful predictors, although not as good as TPSA. The predictive value of the SII for PCA and CSPCa is not excellent.

In addition, we also used the Delong test to compare the diagnostic efficacy of TPSA +PIV compared with using TPSA alone for PCa/CSPCa. The diagnostic efficacy of TPSA + PIV (AUC = 0.700, 95% CI: 0.642–0.757) for PCa is higher than that of TPSA (AUC = 0.657, 95% CI: 0.596–0.717) with a statistical difference (p = 0.02).

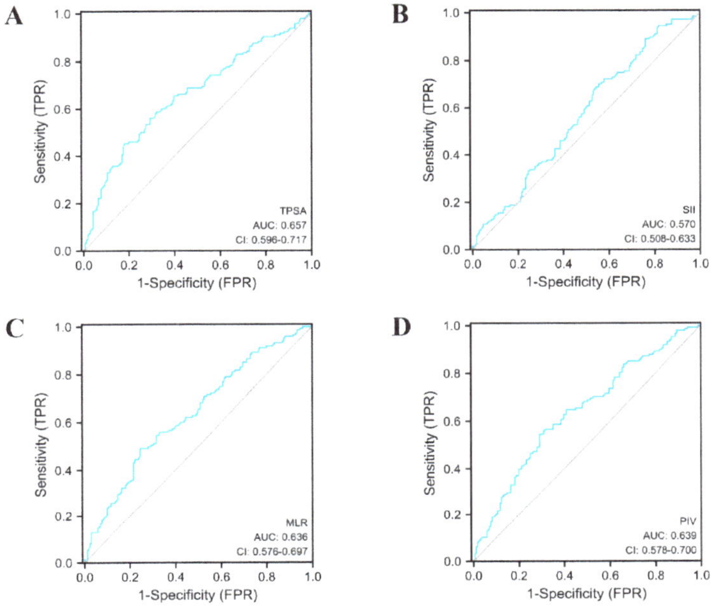

Figure 2. The AUC curves of TPSA and inflammatory markers in prostate cancer. (**A**): The AUC curves of TPSA; (**B**): The AUC curves of SII; (**C**): The AUC curves of MLR; (**D**): The AUC curves of PIV.

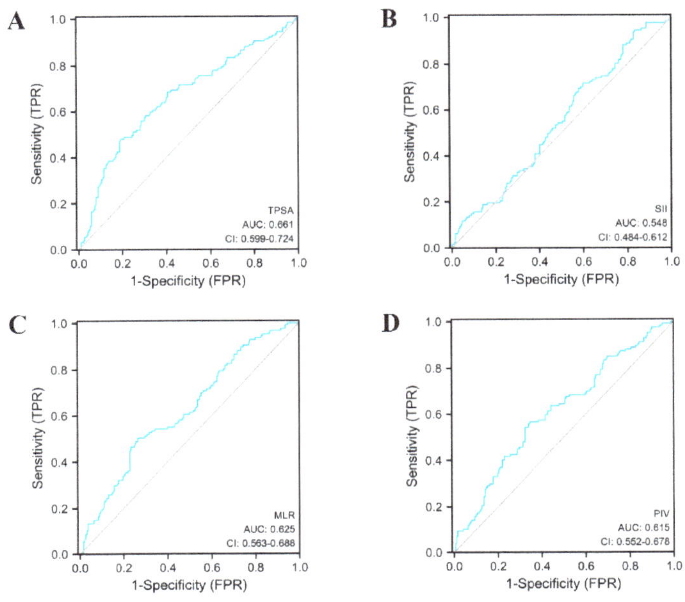

Figure 3. The AUC curves of TPSA and inflammatory markers in clinically significant prostate cancer. (**A**): The AUC curves of TPSA; (**B**): The AUC curves of SII; (**C**): The AUC curves of MLR; (**D**): The AUC curves of PIV.

3.5. Development of a Nomogram for PCa Prediction

In order to intuitively show the predictive value of the PIV for PCa, we developed a nomogram (Figure 4) for positive biopsy prediction in prostate biopsy patients based on Model C; patients in this study were randomly divided into a training group and validation group according to the random number table in a 3:1 ratio. The calibration curve of the nomogram demonstrated good agreement between prediction and observation in the training group (Supplementary Figure S1A) and validation group (Supplementary Figure S1B). The decision curve analysis (Supplementary Figure S2) illustrated that the nomogram model has excellent clinical application.

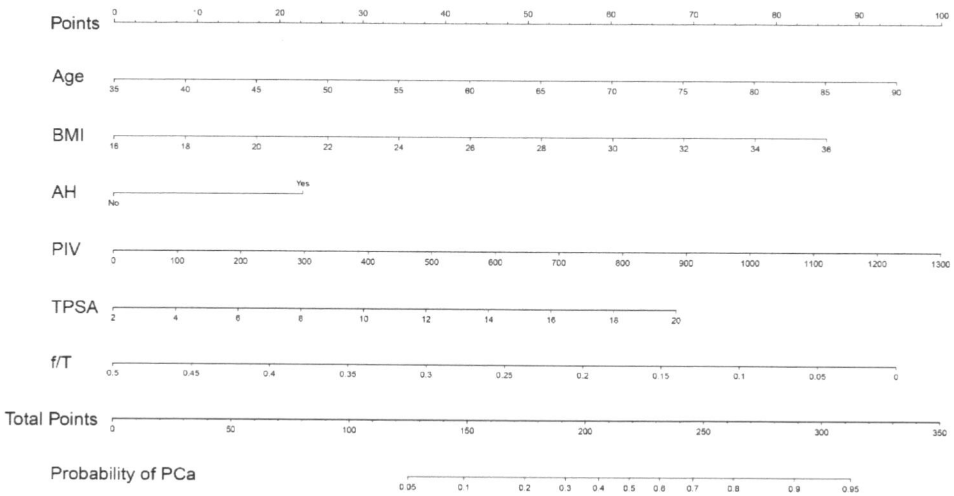

Figure 4. Nomogram for predicting PCa based on the training cohort. The prostate biopsy nomogram was developed in the training cohort, with age, BMI, AH, PIV, TPSA, and f/T incorporated. BMI: body mass index; AH: alcohol history; PIV: pan-immune-inflammation value; TPSA: total prostatic specific antigen; f/T: free/total prostatic specific antigen ratio.

4. Discussion

In this retrospective study of patients undergoing prostate biopsies with PSA values of 4.0–20.0ng/mL, we found that compared with non-PCa patients, the PIV and MLR of the patients with PCa were significantly higher. In addition, the PIV and MLR showed high predictive values in both the univariable prediction models and the multivariable prediction models of PCa and CSPCa. The SII was also significantly elevated in the PCa patients, but there was no significant difference between the CSPCa and Non-CSPCa groups, and its predictive value for PCa and CSPCa was not as good as the MLR and PIV. Meanwhile, other systemic inflammatory markers, such as the NLR, dNLR, and PLR, had limited diagnostic value for PCa and CSPCa.

Inflammation within the tumor microenvironment has effects that promote malignant transformations in cells, as well as carcinogenesis and its progression [10]. Inflammation not only works as a promoter during carcinogenesis (inflammation-induced cancer), but growing tumors that escape immunosurveillance also induce an inflammatory response that can support cancer progression (cancer-related inflammation) [11]. More and more studies show that with the occurrence and progression of cancer, a series of changes will occur in inflammatory-related cells and inflammatory-related substances in patients, which are closely related to the diagnosis and prognosis of tumors, such as the systemic increase in neutrophils [12], elevated levels of circulating monocytes [13], thrombocytosis [14], and lymphopenia [15]. The PIV incorporates the above inflammatory indicators into one equation, and several studies have confirmed that the PIV has a good predictive effect on the prognosis of some tumor patients. Our study explored the diagnostic value of the PIV in PCa for the first time and proved that the PIV is a significant predictor for PCa and CSPCa [8].

A growing number of studies have explored the potential diagnostic value of different kinds of systemic inflammatory indicators in PCa. However, contradictory results were reported from these studies. A retrospective study by Pawel et al. [16] found that the MLR was not helpful for the diagnosis of PCa. Another four studies, including a large retrospective analysis [17–20], showed that the MLR is an important predictor in PCa diagnosis, which is consistent with our findings. In conclusion, we believe that a higher MLR level is significantly related to the detection of PCa/CSPCa. The diagnostic value of the NLR, PLR, and SII for PCa has been controversial. The research of Durvesh [21] and Hiroshi [22] showed that the NLR is a good predictor of PCa, while the research of Du [23] showed that the NLR has a limited diagnostic value for PCa. The conclusions of other studies [16,18,19] are the same as the outcomes of Du's study. Our study showed that the NLR may not be a valuable predictor of PCA/CSPCa. The results of two studies [24,25] pointed out that a higher PLR is related to the detection of PCa, while other studies [16,18,19,26,27] showed that there is no obvious relationship between the PLR and PCa. A similar situation has been found in studies of the SII [16,24,27]. In our study, the PLR has no significance in the diagnosis of PCa; although the SII had a certain diagnostic value for PCa, it is not as good as the PIV and MLR. We believe that the reasons for the above contradictory conclusions may be mainly related to the inconsistent clinical risk stratification of the patients participating in the study. Some studies included low-risk patients with PSA values of 4–10 ng/mL before their biopsies, which means that the changes in the systemic inflammation indicators in these patients may not be obvious, and patients were not grouped according to PSA levels in other studies. In addition, the date of blood sample collection before the biopsies and the method of the biopsies also have a certain impact on the results of the study.

To our knowledge, this study is the first report on the predictive effect of the PIV on PCa. In our study, we compared the superiority of the PIV with that of other systemic inflammatory indices, such as the MLR and SII. Compared with PIV, MLR and SII did not include the neutrophil count × platelet count and monocyte count, respectively. The PIV showed good diagnostic value, both for PCa and CSPCa. After a comprehensive consideration of the patients' age, BMI, history of alcohol use, and TPSA and f/T values, the diagnostic value of the PIV (model C) for PCA/CSPCa is better than that of the MLR (model A) and the SII (model B). The ROC analysis and the result of the prognostic model showed that the PIV was better than the MLR and SII in its comprehensive value regarding the prediction of PCa. It should be noted that the interaction among inflammation, immunity, and cancers is complex and interlocking. The PIV was created to involve more mediators in the immune-inflammatory markers to more accurately model and reflect the inflammatory environment in patients with PCa so that it has better predictive power than incomplete systemic inflammatory indices. In addition, in the comparison of the diagnostic value of TPSA and TPSA + PIV for PCa, the combination of PIV + TPSA (AUC = 0.700, 95CI: 0.642–0.757) was proven to be more significant than TPSA (AUC = 0.657, 95CI: 0.596–0.717) ($p = 0.02$). These findings of this study may have significant clinical implications. This is because, although PSA screening has been widely implemented in decision making for prostate biopsies in clinical practice [28], its low specificity for PCa generally leads to many unnecessary biopsies [29]. According to the results of our study, the PIV, which can be measured easily, was shown to be a feasible index that can be used in any clinical setting. Most importantly, the combination of the PIV and TPSA likely improves the accuracy of prostate biopsies in patients with PSA values of 4.0–20.0 ng/mL, and it may be useful for making better preoperative assessments and individualized treatment decisions. These findings suggest that it is necessary to perform the routine blood tests as a routine test in such patients. In the current study, we chose the PIV, together with age, BMI, history of alcohol use, and TPSA and f/T values to develop a new nomogram to predict PCa risk. Our nomogram had a good potential for discrimination and calibration, which was confirmed by the internal validation. Unfortunately, we did not conduct an independent external validation due to the research conditions.

In addition, we found that higher age, BMI, and alcohol consumption were directly related to the diagnosis of PCa, which was consistent with previous reported results [30–32]. This knowledge could contribute to more efficient risk factor management in populations, which can aid in the prevention of PCa, significantly reducing the impact of this disease on public health.

This study is a single-institution retrospective analysis and therefore has some inherent limitations. Moreover, we did not distinguish between the biopsy strategies because of the limited sample size. Large-scale, multicenter studies are warranted to confirm our findings in the future.

5. Conclusions

Our study shows that the PIV and MLR are significant predictors of PCa and CSPCa diagnoses in patients with PSA levels from 4.0 to 20.0 ng/mL, and they may be useful to avoid unnecessary biopsies or biopsy-related morbidities in real clinical practice. The NLR, dNLR, PLR and SII may have a limited role in predicting PCa or CSPCa.

Supplementary Materials: The following are available online at https://www.mdpi.com/article/10.3390/jcm12030820/s1, Figure S1: Calibration curves of the nomogram for PCa detection in the training, and validation cohorts, Figure S2: Decision curve analysis of the nomogram for PCa detection.

Author Contributions: M.Z. and Y.Z. (Yongheng Zhou) performed the data analyses and wrote the manuscript. Z.L., Z.J., W.Q., S.C. and W.W. participated in the collection of samples and clinical data. B.S. and Y.Z. (Yaofeng Zhu) participated in the study design and revising of the manuscript. All authors have read and agreed to the published version of the manuscript.

Funding: This work was supported by the Natural Science Foundation of Shandong Province (ZR2021MH318 to Y.Z. (Yaofeng Zhu)).

Institutional Review Board Statement: The studies involving human participants were reviewed and approved by Ethical Committee of the Qilu Hospital of Shandong University (KYLL-202111-107).

Informed Consent Statement: Written informed consent for participation was not required for this study in accordance with the institutional requirements and the national legislation.

Data Availability Statement: The original contributions presented in the study are included in the article/Supplementary Material. Further inquiries can be directed to the corresponding author.

Conflicts of Interest: The authors declare that the research was conducted in the absence of any commercial or financial relationships that could be construed as a potential conflict of interest.

References

1. Kang, Y.; Song, P.; Fang, K.; Yang, B.; Yang, L.; Zhou, J.; Wang, L.; Dong, Q. Survival outcomes of low prostate-specific antigen levels and T stages in patients with high-grade prostate cancer: A population-matched study. *J. Cancer* **2020**, *11*, 6484–6490. [CrossRef] [PubMed]
2. Humphrey, P.A.; Andriole, G.L. Prostate cancer diagnosis. *Mo. Med.* **2010**, *107*, 107–112.
3. Ried, K.; Tamanna, T.; Matthews, S.; Eng, P.; Sali, A. New Screening Test Improves Detection of Prostate Cancer Using Circulating Tumor Cells and Prostate-Specific Markers. *Front. Oncol.* **2020**, *10*, 582. [CrossRef] [PubMed]
4. Brikun, I.; Nusskern, D.; Decatus, A.; Harvey, E.; Li, L.; Freije, D. A panel of DNA methylation markers for the detection of prostate cancer from FV and DRE urine DNA. *Clin. Epigenet.* **2018**, *10*, 91. [CrossRef] [PubMed]
5. Nevo, A.; Navaratnam, A.; Andrews, P. Prostate cancer and the role of biomarkers. *Abdom. Radiol.* **2020**, *45*, 2120–2132. [CrossRef] [PubMed]
6. Xie, H.; Ruan, G.; Ge, Y.; Zhang, Q.; Zhang, H.; Lin, S.; Song, M.; Zhang, X.; Liu, X.; Li, X.; et al. Inflammatory burden as a prognostic biomarker for cancer. *Clin. Nutr.* **2022**, *41*, 1236–1243. [CrossRef]
7. Mullally, W.J.; Greene, J.; Jordan, E.J.; Horgan, A.M.; O'Connor, M.; Calvert, P.M. The prognostic value of the derived neutrophil-to-lymphocyte ratio (dNLR) in patients treated with immune checkpoint inhibitors. *Ir. J. Med. Sci.* **2022**. [CrossRef] [PubMed]
8. Guven, D.C.; Sahin, T.K.; Erul, E.; Kilickap, S.; Gambichler, T.; Aksoy, S. The Association between the Pan-Immune-Inflammation Value and Cancer Prognosis: A Systematic Review and Meta-Analysis. *Cancers* **2022**, *14*, 2675. [CrossRef]

9. Barakzai, M.A. Prostatic Adenocarcinoma: A Grading from Gleason to the New Grade-Group System: A Historical and Critical Review. *Asian Pac. J. Cancer Prev.* **2019**, *20*, 661–666. [CrossRef]
10. Mantovani, A.; Allavena, P.; Sica, A.; Balkwill, F. Cancer-related inflammation. *Nature* **2008**, *454*, 436–444. [CrossRef]
11. Coussens, L.M.; Zitvogel, L.; Palucka, A.K. Neutralizing tumor-promoting chronic inflammation: A magic bullet? *Science* **2013**, *339*, 286–291. [CrossRef] [PubMed]
12. Powell, D.R.; Huttenlocher, A. Neutrophils in the Tumor Microenvironment. *Trends Immunol.* **2016**, *37*, 41–52. [CrossRef] [PubMed]
13. Engblom, C.; Pfirschke, C.; Pittet, M.J. The role of myeloid cells in cancer therapies. *Nat. Rev. Cancer* **2016**, *16*, 447–462. [CrossRef] [PubMed]
14. Haemmerle, M.; Stone, R.L.; Menter, D.G.; Afshar-Kharghan, V.; Sood, A.K. The Platelet Lifeline to Cancer: Challenges and Opportunities. *Cancer Cell* **2018**, *33*, 965–983. [CrossRef]
15. Ray-Coquard, I.; Cropet, C.; Van Glabbeke, M.; Sebban, C.; Le Cesne, A.; Judson, I.; Tredan, O.; Verweij, J.; Biron, P.; Labidi, I.; et al. Lymphopenia as a prognostic factor for overall survival in advanced carcinomas, sarcomas, and lymphomas. *Cancer Res.* **2009**, *69*, 5383–5391. [CrossRef] [PubMed]
16. Rajwa, P.; Huebner, N.A.; Hostermann, D.I.; Grossmann, N.C.; Schuettfort, V.M.; Korn, S.; Quhal, F.; König, F.; Mostafaei, H.; Laukhtina, E.; et al. Evaluation of the Predictive Role of Blood-Based Biomarkers in the Context of Suspicious Prostate MRI in Patients Undergoing Prostate Biopsy. *J. Pers. Med.* **2021**, *11*, 1231. [CrossRef]
17. Cho, M.C.; Yoo, S.; Choo, M.S.; Son, H.; Jeong, H. Lymphocyte-to-monocyte ratio is a predictor of clinically significant prostate cancer at prostate biopsy. *Prostate* **2021**, *81*, 1278–1286. [CrossRef]
18. Caglayan, V.; Onen, E.; Avci, S.; Sambel, M.; Kilic, M.; Oner, S.; Aydos, M.M.; Yıldız, H.E. Lymphocyte-to-monocyte ratio is a valuable marker to predict prostate cancer in patients with prostate specific antigen between 4 and 10 ng/dl. *Arch. Ital. Urol. Androl* **2019**, *90*, 270–275. [CrossRef]
19. Hou, G.-D.; Zheng, Y.; Zheng, W.-X.; Gao, M.; Zhang, L.; Hou, N.-N.; Yuan, J.R.; Wei, D.; Ju, D.E.; Dun, X.L.; et al. A novel nomogram predicting the risk of positive biopsy for patients in the diagnostic gray area of prostate cancer. *Sci. Rep.* **2020**, *10*, 17675. [CrossRef]
20. Zhou, Z.H.; Liu, F.; Wang, W.J.; Liu, X.; Sun, L.J.; Zhu, Y.; Ye, D.W.; Zhang, G.M. Development and validation of a nomogram including lymphocyte-to-monocyte ratio for initial prostate biopsy: A double-center retrospective study. *Asian J. Androl.* **2021**, *23*, 41–46. [CrossRef]
21. Jethwani, D.L.; Sivamoorthy, L.L. Toh, C.C.; Malek, R. Predicting the diagnosis of prostate cancer with a scoring system based on novel biomarkers. *BMC Urol.* **2022**, *22*, 13. [CrossRef] [PubMed]
22. Masuda, H.; Mikami, K.; Otsuka, K.; Hou, K.; Suyama, T.; Araki, K.; Kojima, S.; Naya, Y. Validation of the Effectiveness of Neutrophil-to-lymphocyte Ratio (NLR) as a Predictive Factor in Patients Undergoing Prostate Biopsy With Prostate Specific Antigen (PSA) Between 4.0 and 10.0 ng/mL. *In Vivo* **2021**, *35*, 1641–1646. [CrossRef]
23. Du, J.; Lim, E.J.; Huang, H.H.; Lau, W.K.O. Predictive value of neutrophil-to-lymphocyte ratio in diagnosis of early prostate cancer among men who underwent robotic transperineal prostate biopsy. *Medicine* **2021**, *100*, e28007. [CrossRef] [PubMed]
24. Sonmez, G.; Demirtas, T.; Tombul, S.T.; Akgun, H.; Demirtas, A. Diagnostic efficiency of systemic immune-inflammation index in fusion prostate biopsy. *Actas Urol. Esp. Engl. Ed.* **2021**, *45*, 359–365. [CrossRef] [PubMed]
25. Adhyatma, K.P.; Warli, S.M. Diagnostic Value of Platelet-To-Lymphocyte Ratio in Prostate Cancer. *Open Access Maced. J. Med. Sci.* **2019**, *7*, 1093–1096. [CrossRef]
26. Lee, J.W.; Jeong, H.; Son, H.; Cho M.C. Platelet-to-lymphocyte ratio is not a predictor of clinically significant prostate cancer at the prostate biopsy: A large cohort study. *Sci. Rep.* **2021**, *11*, 14240. [CrossRef]
27. Murray, N.P.; Fuentealba, C.; Salazar, A.; Reyes, E. Platelet-to-lymphocyte ratio and systemic immune-inflammation index versus circulating prostate cells to predict significant prostate cancer at first biopsy. *Turk. J. Urol.* **2020**, *46*, 115–122. [CrossRef]
28. Huang, D.; Yang, X.; Wu, Y.; Lin, X.; Xu, D.; Na, R.; Xu, J. Cost-Effectiveness Analysis of Prostate Health Index in Decision Making for Initial Prostate Biopsy. *Front. Oncol.* **2020**, *10*, 565382. [CrossRef]
29. Chen, N.; Rong, M.; Shao, X.; Zhang, H.; Liu, S.; Dong, B.; Xue, W.; Wang, T.; Li, T.; Pan, J. Surface-enhanced Raman spectroscopy of serum accurately detects prostate cancer in patients with prostate-specific antigen levels of 4-10 ng/mL. *Int. J. Nanomed.* **2017**, *12*, 5399–5407. [CrossRef]
30. Perez-Cornago, A.; Appleby, P.N. Pischon, T.; Tsilidis, K.K.; Tjonneland, A.; Olsen, A.; Overvad, K.; Kaaks, R.; Kühn, T.; Boeing, H.; et al. Tall height and obesity are associated with an increased risk of aggressive prostate cancer: Results from the EPIC cohort study. *BMC Med.* **2017**, *15*, 115. [CrossRef]

31. Bray, F.; Ferlay, J.; Soerjomataram, I.; Siegel, R.L.; Torre, L.A.; Jemal, A. Global cancer statistics 2018: GLOBOCAN estimates of incidence and mortality worldwide for 36 cancers in 185 countries. *CA Cancer J. Clin.* **2018**, *68*, 394–424. [CrossRef] [PubMed]
32. Bagnardi, V.; Rota, M.; Botteri, E.; Tramacere, I.; Islami, F.; Fedirko, V.; Scotti, L.; Jenab, M.; Turati, F.; Pasquali, E.; et al. Alcohol consumption and site-specific cancer risk: A comprehensive dose-response meta-analysis. *Br. J. Cancer* **2015**, *112*, 580–593. [CrossRef] [PubMed]

Journal of
Clinical Medicine

MDPI

Review

A Review of Modern Imaging Landscape for Prostate Cancer: A Comprehensive Clinical Guide

Paul Gravestock [1], Bhaskar Kumar Somani [2], Theodoros Tokas [3,4] and Bhavan Prasad Rai [1,*]

1 Department of Urology, Freeman Hospital, Newcastle upon Tyne NE7 7DN, UK
2 Department of Urology, University Hospital Southampton NHS Trust, Southampton SO16 6YD, UK
3 Department of Urology and Andrology, General Hospital Hall in Tirol, 6060 Hall in Tirol, Austria
4 Training and Research in Urological Surgery and Technology (T.R.U.S.T.)-Group, 6060 Hall in Tirol, Austria
* Correspondence: urobhavan@gmail.com

Abstract: The development of prostate cancer imaging is rapidly evolving, with many changes to the way patients are diagnosed, staged, and monitored for recurrence following treatment. New developments, including the potential role of imaging in screening and the combined diagnostic and therapeutic applications in the field of theranostics, are underway. In this paper, we aim to outline the current landscape in prostate cancer imaging and look to the future at the potential modalities and applications to come.

Keywords: prostatic neoplasms; image-guided biopsy; multiparametric magnetic resonance imaging; positron-emission tomography

1. Introduction

Imaging for prostate cancer has developed significantly over the last two decades. There has been a range of modalities utilized, including the recent application of functional imaging. Additionally, indications for imaging have expanded beyond diagnostics to biopsy guidance, staging and risk stratification, active surveillance, and the detection of recurrence. Furthermore, there are developing roles for imaging in population screening and theranostic applications. We aim to provide an up-to-date narrative looking at the role of prostate cancer imaging in these key areas.

2. Imaging in Prostate Cancer Diagnostics

Historically, prostate cancer has been difficult to detect and biopsy. Digital rectal examination (DRE) was the mainstay of diagnosis, with transrectal biopsies targeting palpable lesions [1]. This blind approach was superseded by the development of transrectal ultrasound (TRUS). TRUS utilizes a rectal ultrasound probe to directly visualize the prostate. However, whilst prostate cancer can appear hypoechoic on an ultrasound, it is not an accurate detection method, and as a diagnostic or staging modality, it performs poorly [2,3]. As a result, systematic prostate biopsies in patients with suspected prostate cancer using TRUS to guide the needle became the diagnostic standard. These were initially performed using a sextant biopsy protocol that involved taking three biopsy cores from each side of the prostate. Due to high false negative rates, this was refined to what is termed an extended protocol involving 10–12 total cores, which was found to have an increased sensitivity for prostate cancer detection [4]. However, systematic biopsies that are performed based on DRE findings or prostate specific antigen (PSA) levels do not discriminate well between clinically significant and clinically insignificant cancers. One tool that has been subsequently introduced to improve diagnostic accuracy is multiparametric MRI (mpMRI).

mpMRI has been shown to be highly sensitive in the diagnosis of prostate cancer. The PROMIS trial found mpMRI to have a sensitivity of 93%, estimating that its introduction into the diagnostic pathway would avoid up to 27% of patients undergoing an initial prostate biopsy and result in fewer clinically insignificant cancer diagnoses [5]. It has subsequently become the first line imaging used in the diagnosis of localized prostate cancer, with patients found to have a raised PSA level or abnormal DRE routinely undergoing mpMRI prior to prostate biopsy [6]. mpMRI consists of a combination of MRI sequences; anatomical sequences providing detail of the prostate, in particular T2-weighted (T2W) images, and functional sequences including diffusion weighted imaging (DWI) and dynamic contrast enhancement (DCE), to assess for features suspicious for potential prostate cancer [7]. The interpretation is standardized, using either the Prostate Imaging-Reporting and Data System (PI-RADS) or Likert scoring systems that aim to quantify the likelihood of clinically significant prostate cancer being present on a scale of 1 to 5 [7,8].

There is ongoing debate in the relation to mpMRI for prostate cancer diagnostics regarding the use of DCE, and to whether T2W and DWI alone, termed biparametric MRI (bpMRI), is sufficient. bpMRI has been shown to be non-inferior to mpMRI and has the advantage of being less time-consuming while removing the risk associated with contrast media, though at present there remains no clear consensus [9–12].

2.1. Screening

Prostate cancer screening itself is a contentious issue. Screening using PSA has been examined by several large trials. The CAP trial in the United Kingdom (UK) examined prostate cancer screening in over 400,000 men who underwent a single PSA test ± biopsy when raised and found no significant difference in prostate cancer mortality between those who underwent PSA screening and the control arm at 10 years [13]. The European Randomized Study of Screening for Prostate Cancer (ERSPC) followed up with over 180,000 men undergoing regular PSA screening (between two and seven yearly intervals) with biopsies if raised and found that prostate cancer mortality was reduced in the screened arm. However, this was associated with a high number needed to diagnose of 1 in 48 to avert one prostate cancer death at a follow-up of 9 years, though this was reduced to 1 in 18 at 16 years showing an increased benefit with a longer follow-up [14]. Despite this improvement in mortality that is seen with PSA screening, it comes at the cost of considerable overdiagnosis, and potential overtreatment, of clinically insignificant prostate cancer.

As discussed previously, mpMRI has been shown to reduce the number of clinically insignificant cancers diagnosed, and on this basis, screening using an MRI has been investigated. In the IP1-PROSTAGRAM trial, 408 men underwent a PSA, MRI, and TRUS (B-mode and shear wave elastography); men who were deemed to be positive in any of the three tests (reporters of imaging were blinded to PSA) underwent a systematic transperineal (TP) biopsy + targeted cores if they were found to be positive at MRI or TRUS. In this trial, MRI was found to detect more clinically significant and less clinically insignificant cancers than PSA alone [15]. Other trials are in progress further examining this. ReIMAGINE is a study assessing screening for prostate cancer within a UK population, randomly inviting around 300 eligible men aged 50–75 for an MRI to assess the feasibility of screening and prevalence of MRI-detected suspicious lesions in the general population, for which recruitment was completed in December 2020 [16]. Additionally, MRI vs. PSA (MVP) is a Canadian randomized controlled trial awaiting publication that compares men undergoing screening via PSA with a subsequent biopsy if raised vs. those screened with an MRI and followed up by US-MRI fusion biopsy if abnormal lesions are detected [17]. Of note, all three of the above trials used bpMRI.

2.2. Biopsies

Prostate biopsies are used to further assess patients with suspicious mpMRI results in the context of other factors, such as PSA and DRE findings. Biopsies were predominately undertaken by a transrectal (TR) approach, though more recently, there has been a shift toward TP biopsies. This has been driven by an increasing body of evidence showing lower infectious complications and a reduced antibiotic prophylaxis requirement for TP biopsies, with some studies suggesting that, in select patients, no antibiotic prophylaxis is required at all [18–22]. As a result, this is reflected in international guidance with the European Association of Urology (EAU) guidance, which strongly recommends using a TP approach [6]. Additionally, TRANSLATE is a randomized control trial (RCT) looking to definitively address which approach is better, directly comparing local anaesthetic (LA) TP prostate biopsy with LA TR prostate biopsy. The primary outcome evaluated will be the detection of clinically significant prostate cancer, with secondary outcomes including infection rates, tolerability, complications, cost effectiveness, and the need for repeated biopsies [23].

Prostate biopsies can be used to target suspicious MRI lesions or systematically sample the prostate. The PRECISION trial showed that when men with a clinical suspicion for prostate cancer underwent mpMRI followed by targeted biopsies, there was a higher detection rate for clinically significant prostate cancer and less clinically insignificant prostate cancers detected than those who underwent indiscriminate systematic biopsies [24]. Further studies, including 4M, MRI-FIRST, and PAIREDCAP, have shown that the best detection rates are achieved by combining systematic and targeted biopsies with the omission of either set shown to miss a proportion of clinically significant cancers. For example, in patients undergoing MR-targeted biopsies, the addition of systematic biopsies yielded the detection of 7% extra clinically significant cancers in the 4M trial and 5.2% in MRI-First. As a result, a combined approach is recommended [6,25–27]. Key trials examining mpMRI- and MR-targeted biopsies (TB) that were compared with systematic biopsies (SB) are summarized in Table 1.

Transrectal ultrasound allow for the visualization of the prostate anatomy and the biopsy needle, usually in both the axial and sagittal planes. Targeted biopsies can be performed using a cognitive approach whereby the operator reviews the MRI imaging and estimates the corresponding area on TRUS imaging. Alternatively, fusion software can be used to directly superimpose the suspicious areas seen on the MRI over the TRUS images. Novel robotic solutions have been developed in conjunction with fusion software to increase targeting accuracy. These include systems that use a robotic needle guide to target the suspicious lesion, defining the position and depth with the operating surgeon only required to insert the biopsy gun and fire [28].

The limitations of fusion-guided biopsies are primarily related to the process of accurately overlaying the MRI targets onto the live TRUS images, thereby methods have been developed to cut out the TRUS middleman in the form of in-bore MRI biopsies [29]. An in-bore MRI biopsy involves a rectal needle guide and sequential MRI imaging with the patient removed from the scanner and the needle guide adjusted, with further MRI sequences performed until it is adequately aligned with the area of interest. At this point, the patient can be removed from the scanner and a biopsy can be taken, with the option for confirmatory re-imaging if required [30]. Again, novel robotic solutions have been developed to streamline this process; these include systems that utilize pneumatic stepper motors powered by compressed air (in order to remain MRI compatible) to adjust a needle guide from within the control room, thereby removing the need for the patient to be removed from the scanner and the needle guide manually adjusted between each set of images [31,32].

Table 1. Summary of key trials examining mpMRI is prostate cancer diagnosis/biopsy.

							Clinically Significant Cancer			Clinically Insignificant Cancer	
	Year		**Design**	**Cohort Size**		**Clinically Significant Definition**	**MRI [a] Sensitivity**	**TRUS [b] Biopsy Sensitivity**			
PROMIS [5]	2017	Biopsy Naive	All men, MRI + TRUS + TP [c] Grid	576		Gleason score ≥ 4 + 3 or cancer containing core ≥ 6 mm	93%	48%			
				MRI TB [d]	**SB**		**MRI TB Detection Rates**	**SB [e] Detection Rate**	**Combined Detection Rate**	**MRI TB Detection Rates**	**SB Detection Rate**
PRECISION [24]	2018	Biopsy Naive	RCT [f]	252	248		38%	26%		9%	22%
MRI-FIRST [25]	2019	Biopsy Naive	SB + TB (cognitive or US fusion)	275		Gleason score ≥ 3 + 4	32.3%	29.9%	37.5%		
PAIREDCAP [26]	2019	Biopsy Naive	SB + TB (Cognitive and US [g] Fusion)	248		Gleason score ≥ 3 + 4	62.1%	60.1%	70.2%	24%	23%
4M [27]	2019	Biopsy Naive	SB + TB (MRI in-bore)	626		Gleason score ≥ 3 + 4	25%	23%		28%	25%

[a] Magnetic Resonance Imaging, [b] Transrectal Ultrasound [c] Transperineal [d] Targeted Biopsies, [e] Systematic biopsies, [f] Randomized controlled trial [g] Ultrasound.

The FUTURE trial compared cognitive, fusion, and in-bore MRI biopsy techniques in men with prior negative systematic biopsies and an ongoing suspicion of prostate cancer and found no difference in detection rates, though it was underpowered [33]. Other evidence is differing with no clear consensus on the best modality. Therefore, in-bore MRI biopsies do not currently seem to sufficiently justify the cost implications of the associated additional MRI time [34–36]. Though limited, initial evidence suggests that robot-assisted MRI-US fusion transperineal-targeted biopsies may have higher cancer detection rates and lower complications than cognitive-guided transperineal biopsies [28].

2.3. PET Imaging in Diagnosis

Molecular imaging in the form of positron emission tomography (PET) scanning has been used in the field of prostate cancer for some time. PET uses different radiolabelled tracers to identify and target specific biological pathways with a wide range and an increasing number of applications [37]. Radiolabels are positron-emitters; the emission of a positron leads to a positron-electron annihilation and subsequent production of two annihilation photons travelling in opposite directions. The annihilation photons can then be captured by the ring of detectors within the PET scanner. Conventional PET images have a resolution of around 4–5 mm and, as such, are usually performed in combination with a higher resolution modality to provide more detailed anatomical information, typically computed tomography (CT) [38].

Diagnostic accuracy in PET is dependent on the radiotracer used, with different tracers appropriate in different applications. In prostate cancer, several radiotracers have been trialled, including Choline, Fluciclovine, and prostate-specific membrane antigen (PSMA) [37]. Choline PET/CT, for example, has been studied in the primary diagnosis of prostate cancer, though it was seen to produce high rates of false negative and false positive results due to poor uptake in some tumours and excessive uptake in benign prostate tissue, with sensitivity and specificity in one study found to be 66% and 81%, respectively [39,40]. However, PSMA is a membrane-bound glycoprotein expressed predominately on prostate epithelial cells and shows increased expression in prostate cancer [41,42].

Whilst PSMA is primarily found within the prostate gland, its expression elsewhere has become increasingly recognized with the potential for false positives. It can be found in the vascular endothelium (and to a lesser extent, the tumour cells) of a number of other primary malignancies, which include other adenocarcinomas (breast, colorectal, pancreatic, and gastric), renal cell carcinoma, non-small cell lung cancer, glioblastoma multiforme, and transitional cell carcinoma [43]. Its presence can also be found in a range of normal tissue, such as the salivary glands, kidneys, bowel, spleen, and liver. Additionally, benign conditions, such as sarcoidosis or Paget's disease and benign lesions, including meningiomas or haemangiomas, have been shown to cause false positive results [44,45]. In contrast, PSMA is not expressed in the same way in neuroendocrine prostate cancer, an aggressive variant of the disease, which can lead to false negatives [44].

Another consideration is the effect of androgen deprivation therapy (ADT) on PSMA expression. The effect of ADT appears to be dependent on the type of disease and scan timing, though there are some mixed results. Studies have shown a positive association between ADT use and tumour detection in the setting of recurrent disease [46]. In patients with castrate resistance metastatic disease, an increase in PSMA uptake following ADT commencement has been reported in multiple studies as variable but more pronounced within bony metastases [47,48]. Other studies looking at the treatment of hormone naïve patients with PSMA imaging at longer intervals of around 3 months post ADT have shown a reduction in tracer uptake, presumably corresponding with treatment effect [49,50].

PSMA is commonly targeted using PSMA-11 ligand in combination with the radionucleotide gallium-68 (Ga^{68}-PSMA-11), which has a half-life of 67.7 min [37]. Along with the ^{11}C-Choline and ^{18}F-Fluciclovine radiotracers, it has an established role in the re-staging of patients with a biochemical relapse as part of a PET/CT. However, more recently, PSMA has been investigated in combination with mpMRI as a means of diagnostic imaging. The use of mpMRI over CT has the advantage of the improved anatomical differentiation and the ability to correlate radiotracer uptake with functional MRI sequences, such as DWI. The evidence comparing imaging results and pathology has shown that PSMA PET/MRI has superior diagnostic performance and tumour localization over mpMRI or PSMA PET alone, suggesting that its use as an additional diagnostic parameter is justified [51–56]. When used to target prostatic biopsies, a recent systematic review has shown that PSMA-PET (in combination with either CT or MRI) had a comparable diagnostic accuracy to mpMRI-targeted biopsies with a trend toward increased accuracy when mpMRI and PSMA-PET was used in combination, though it was limited by the lack of available evidence [57].

PRIMARY, a prospective Phase II trial, enrolled 291 biopsy naïve men with suspected prostate cancer. Participants underwent pelvic PSMA PET/CT and mpMRI, followed by systematic and targeted TP biopsy. It found that PSMA PET/CT combined with mpMRI had a higher negative predictive value and sensitivity than mpMRI alone, 91% vs. 72% and 97% vs. 83%, respectively [58]. A follow-up on the Phase III trial, PRIMARY2, is currently recruiting and aims to look at the men with a negative or equivocal MRI. In PRIMARY2, men will be randomized to either pelvic PSMA PET/CT with targeted biopsies if positive, or no biopsies if negative. This will be compared to the current standard of care of no additional imaging and template biopsy [59].

In renal cell carcinoma, it is commonplace for suspicious lesions on imaging to be treated with radical surgery without pathological confirmation. This is in part due to the high level of diagnostic accuracy of CT and a less acceptable non-diagnostic rate/negative predictive value associated with biopsy [60]. With increasing accuracy in diagnostic prostate imaging, it seems we may be nearing an era where proceeding directly to prostatectomy could be considered in select patients.

3. Role of Imaging in Active Surveillance

Low/intermediate-risk prostate cancer can be managed with active surveillance (AS) [6,61]. AS is a monitoring strategy whereby patients undergo a combination of regular physical examination, biochemical monitoring, and, when indicated, repeated mpMRI imaging and/or biopsies, with a view to definitive treatment should the disease progress. This allows patients to avoid or defer the associated morbidity definitive treatment brings, maintaining their quality of life, and it is associated with excellent long-term cancer-specific survival rates [62,63]. Active surveillance follow-up protocols vary. In the UK, the National Institute for Clinical Excellence (NICE) recommend PSA to be checked every 3–4 months in the first year and six monthly thereafter, with annual digital rectal examinations and a repeat MRI at 12–18 months with further MRIs and/or repeated biopsies indicated by concerning examination features or PSA kinetics [61].

mpMRI is used in active surveillance to assess for the progression of the disease in comparison with the baseline diagnostic MRI. This can be assessed formally using the Prostate Cancer Radiological Estimation of Change in Sequential Evaluation (PRECISE) criteria [64]. The PRECISE criteria aims to score the likelihood of disease progression on a scale of 1–5, where 1 or 2 represent disease regression, 3 is a stable disease, and 4 or 5 are varying degrees of radiological progression, with evidence showing that it performs well with a high specificity and positive predictive value (PPV) [64,65].

Previously, AS relied heavily on clinical examination and serial PSA to determine the need for re-biopsy. The relatively recent introduction of mpMRI potentially offers a less invasive alternative if it allows for biopsies to be omitted. However, two recent systematic reviews suggest that omitting biopsies and relying on mpMRI alone has insufficient diagnostic accuracy to exclude disease progression even when studies utilized the PRECISE criteria with a sensitivity and NPV for disease progression of 59–61% and 81–88%, respectively. Although, in one review, the use of the PRECISE criteria showed a non-significant trend toward improved performance [66,67]. That being said, when a reassuring mpMRI is combined with other contextualizing factors such as stable PSA kinetics and, in particular, a low PSA density (<0.15 ng/mL/cm^3), there is evidence to suggest it may allow for repeated biopsies to be safely omitted [68].

Emerging methods to safely reduce repeated biopsies during active surveillance include the use of PSMA PET/CT. Current data on this application is limited, but one study has shown potential to reduce false positives and improve negative predictive value (NPV) compared with mpMRI [69].

4. Radiological Staging in Prostate Cancer

Prostate cancer is staged using the Tumour, Node, Metastasis (TNM) system, which assesses disease across each of its three criteria. It is used alongside PSA levels and histological grade to risk stratify disease and determine appropriate treatments.

Tumour (T) is assessed based on DRE findings, where T1 is impalpable, T2 is confined within the prostate, T3 extends beyond the prostate capsule, and T4 is an invasion into adjacent structures [6]. Whilst the T stage assessment is primarily clinical, it can also be assessed using mpMRI, which has been shown to be highly specific but only moderately sensitive for extraprostatic extension (T3a) and seminal vesicle invasion (T3b) [70,71]. Though MRI has limited sensitivity for picking up these adverse features, where found they have useful implications in their association with an increased risk of biochemical recurrence post-radical prostatectomy [72–74]. Traditionally, the risk of recurrence following definitive treatment was calculated using tools such as Partin's tables. These allow for a risk assessment based on PSA, the clinical stage, and the Gleason score, and the evidence suggests the addition of the MRI into this assessment increases its accuracy [73,75]. An accurate assessment of risk preoperatively is important as it can lead to changes in surgical approach, such as the appropriate avoidance of nerve-sparing techniques to maximize oncological outcomes. However, whether the routine use of pre-operative staging mpMRI improves oncological outcomes in practice is unclear with conflicting evidence at present [76–78].

Nodal staging is assessed based on whether regional lymph node (LN) metastasis is present (N1) or not (N0), with non-regional lymph nodes upstaging to M1a [6]. Metastases are classified by the absence (M0) or presence (M1) of distant metastases, further stratified based on location with M1a assigned for non-regional lymph nodes, M1b for bony metastases, and M1c for metastases for other sites.

Patients at high risk of advanced disease are traditionally assessed with a combination of contrast CT of the abdomen and pelvis, primarily to identify nodal metastasis and technetium 99 (Tc^{99}) bone scan, which examines for bone metastases by way of the increased radiotracer uptake in areas of high bone turnover. However, an accurate assessment of regional lymph nodes using conventional imaging is poor, with both CT and MRI having a low sensitivity of LN metastasis of 42% and 39%, respectively [79]. Additionally, whilst Tc^{99} bone scans are sensitive for bone turnover, this can lead to false positives and has the potential to miss early metastasis [80]. Although specificity can be increased with the addition of Single Photo Emission Computed Tomography (SPECT), alternative methods, such as whole-body MRI and PET/CT, have been shown to be superior in the detection of bony metastasis [81–83]. In a systematic review by Zhou et al., PSMA-PET/CT was found to have the highest sensitivity and specificity (97% & 100%) compared with whole-body MRIs (91% & 96%) or bone scintigraphy (86% & 95%) for detecting bone metastases on a per-patient basis [84]. More recently, a large RCT, proPSMA compared conventional imaging (CT and bone scan) with Ga^{68}-PSMA-11 PET/CT and found the latter to have a higher sensitivity (85% vs. 38%) and specificity (98% vs. 91%) for the detection of a pelvic nodal or distant metastases [85]. Furthermore, a more recent Phase 2/3 trial OSPREY evaluated the diagnostic accuracy of 18F-DCFPyL-PSMA positron emission tomography/computerized tomography for pelvic lymph node involvement in 252 men undergoing a radical prostatectomy with extended pelvic lymph node dissection. They reported a sensitivity and specificity of 40% and 98%, respectively, though this improved to 60% and 97.9% for nodes >5 mm [86].

Accurate nodal staging is important as patients with N1M0 disease have a high risk of recurrence and, therefore, should be considered for adjuvant therapies dependent on nodal volume [6,87]. Despite the advances in imaging described above, extended pelvic lymph node dissection (ePLND) during radical prostatectomy remains the gold standard of local nodal staging, though this comes at the cost of a higher morbidity compared with a limited dissection [88]. ePLND and PSMA PET/CT have been directly compared with the former found to be significantly more sensitive [89]. Whilst it may not obviate the need for ePLND, predictive models using MRI, along with other factors, have been used to help select out which patients require ePLND [90]. Similar studies using PSMA PET/CT have shown that, combined with low-risk features, it can help avoid ePLND. However, a negative PSMA PET/CT in the high-risk group still necessitates the procedure [91].

Potential novel applications of PSMA imaging include radioguided surgery utilizing preoperative PSMA PET/MRI and intraoperative gamma probe to target avid lesions directly during robot-assisted radical prostatectomy [92]. Whilst extended lymph node dissections have been shown to have little oncological benefit, this technology presents a way to potentially increase accuracy whilst minimizing morbidity [88,92].

PSMA PET/CT's routine use in the staging pathway is likely to increase the cohort of patients who have pelvic nodal and/or low volume metastasis (often termed oligometastatic disease), owing to its increased sensitivity in these patients. The treatment pathway for these patients is unclear, particularly regarding the role of localized treatment i.e., prostate radiotherapy or radical prostatectomy—often termed cytoreductive prostatectomy in this context. Current available evidence includes subgroup analyses from arms of the STAMPEDE trial, which examined the benefit of local prostate radiotherapy for patients with metastatic prostate cancer. Whilst no difference in overall survival was observed with the addition of radiotherapy, in a subgroup analyses looking only at patients with low-volume disease (low metastatic burden defined as less than four bones and no visceral metastases) a significant survival benefit was observed: 81% vs. 73% at 3 years [93]. There are a number of smaller retrospective studies examining the role of cytoreductive prostatectomy or radical radiotherapy in metastatic prostate cancer, and a recent systematic review examining these found that cytoreductive prostatectomy was associated with a significantly higher overall survival than systematic therapy (OR 2.54 at 5 years) and which was comparable to radiation therapy [94]. The other evidence includes a large population study using Surveillance Epidemiology and End Results (SEER) data from 2004–2010, examining the role of brachytherapy or radical prostatectomy in metastatic disease, which showed an increased survival in patients undergoing these treatments compared with those receiving no surgery or radiotherapy [95].

Further high-quality evidence is required to help further define the role of PSMA PET/CT in staging and the appropriate treatment for the low-volume metastatic prostate cancer cohort. The TROMBONE prospective randomized feasibility trial assessed radical prostatectomy for patients with oligometastatic disease and found that an RCT in this context is feasible. A number of trials are being conducted in this area at present. IP2-ATLANTA is one such RCT in progress, comparing the standard of care to a minimally invasive ablative therapy, cytoreductive prostatectomy, or radiotherapy [96,97].

5. Detection of Recurrent Disease

Recurrence following definitive treatment is typically monitored using PSA. In instances where recurrence has been noted, biochemically treatment options vary based on the original treatment received and whether the recurrence is visible radiologically. The latter has become increasingly important, with early evidence suggesting a survival benefit in those patients with oligometastatic disease who receive metastasis-directed therapy (MDT), which can include surgery or stereotactic body radiotherapy (SBRT) [98,99]. Early detection is also important with higher rates of curative salvage therapy seen when treatment is undertaken at low PSA levels.

This setting is perhaps the best established for PET/CT imaging. Studies have shown PSMA PET/CT to have a high level of accuracy, as it is able to detect recurrence at lower PSA levels than conventional imaging [86,100,101]. Among these, CONDOR, a Phase III trial, enrolled over 200 men with suspected recurrent prostate cancer and negative or equivocal conventional imaging. It found that PSMA-PET was able to detect a lesion in over 60% of these patients and that almost two-thirds of these patients underwent a change in management as a result [101]. Likewise, the OSPREY trial reported additional presumed metastatic disease in around 58% of patients with 18F-DCFPyL-PSMA PET/CT that conventional imaging was unable to detect in the recurrent setting. Additionally, they reported a sensitivity and specificity of 96% and 82%, respectively, for recurrent disease with 18F-DCFPyL-PSMA PET/CT [86]. There have been a number of recent systematic reviews performed to assess diagnostic performances of PET/CT in the recurrent disease setting. Wang et al. compared detection rates of ^{18}F labelled fluciclovine, choline, and PSMA radiotracers and found PSMA to be better than fluciclovine and choline. This was most pronounced at low PSA levels with detection rates of 58% for PSMA vs. 35% and 23% for choline and fluciclovine, respectively [102]. Other systematic reviews have similarly concluded that PSMA is the superior choice of radiotracer. However, there are several different radiolabels that can be utilized [103–107].

The two most commonly used radiolabels for PSMA are gallium-68 [^{68}Ga] or fluoride-18 [^{18}F] [108,109]. A recent systematic review by Evangelista et al. found limited head-to-head evidence between the two radiolabels but noted a number of factors to take into account. For example, whilst ^{68}Ga has the largest evidence base, it has a short half-life of 68 minutes, which can make distribution difficult unless on site or nearby ^{68}Ga generators are available [110]. Furthermore, it has a high positron energy that may limit resolution, and it is primarily excreted via urine, which can limit the detection of small-volume disease adjacent to the urinary tract. In contrast, ^{18}F has a half-life of 110 min, a low positron energy, and is primarily excreted by the liver, which can improve the detection of locoregional recurrence but may reduce sensitivity for the detection of visceral metastases [110]. Although limited by significant heterogeneity, Ma et al. found in their systematic review looking at detection rates for different radiotracers in recurrent prostate cancer that ^{18}F labelled PSMA had a significantly higher detection rate than ^{68}Ga [103].

The majority of studies focus on the use of PET combined with CT. However, with its role expanding in primary diagnosis, PET/MRI has also been described in the recurrent disease setting where, like PET/CT, it has been shown to have high detection rates and performs well at low levels of PSA [111,112]. However, at present, PET/MRI has not been shown to have superiority over PET/CT in this setting [111,112].

Metastasis Directed Therapy (MDT)

A large proportion of patients who are diagnosed with recurrent prostate cancer after primary treatment do so with a small number of metastases. Whilst they would previously have been treated with surveillance and androgen deprivation therapy, MDT was developed in an effort to treat this cohort more effectively.

Two early randomized trials assessed MDT in men with recurrent prostate cancer with oligometastases. The STOMP trial randomized 62 men to MDT or surveillance. The majority of those receiving MDT underwent SBRT (n = 25), though a small portion underwent salvage lymph node dissection (n = 5), and one patient underwent a visceral metastectomy [98]. A similar study, ORIOLE, randomized 54 men to SBRT (n = 36) or surveillance (n = 18) [113]. Both trials allowed for up to three metastases and measured outcomes as disease progression, though STOMP defined this as time to ADT and ORIOLE as progression based on PSA increase, radiological progression, initiation of ADT, symptomatic progression, or death [98,113]. ORIOLE utilized PSMA PET/CT scans to detect recurrence, whereas a limitation of STOMP is that they used choline PET/CT, which, as previously discussed, is less sensitive at detecting recurrent disease [98,113]. Both studies showed benefit of MDT with pooled long-term outcomes reported showing progression free survival of 11.9 months for the MDT cohort compared with 5.9 for those undergoing surveillance [114].

Further studies examining the role of MDT are underway, and results are awaited to further define the treatment pathway in these patients. These include ADOPT, which a randomized Phase III trial comparing MDT with or without 6 months of concurrent ADT in men with recurrent oligometastatic prostate cancer [115]. In a similar cohort, PEACE V-STORM is a multicentre randomized trial comparing MDT + ADT with or without whole pelvic radiotherapy [116]. Another trial examining an alternative systemic therapy is POSTCARD, which aims to compare SBRT to SBRT in combination with Durvalumab, an immunotherapy that aims to enhance the immune response generated by radiotherapy [117].

6. Theranostics in Prostate Cancer

Theranostics is a relatively new term, the definition of which is varied throughout the literature, with some authors even questioning its use entirely [118]. Nonetheless, its use has become commonplace, and in this context we would define it broadly as a combination of diagnostic and therapeutic interventions, one example of which is PSMA-Targeted radioligand therapy. PET imaging uses radioisotopes that emit positrons and, by virtue of immediate annihilation via interaction with an electron, emits two gamma photons that travel through tissue and are detected by the PET scanner detectors. In contrast, potential therapeutic applications can utilize the absorption of radiation into localized tissue as a form of treatment, therefore requiring short penetration distances, such as those seen with beta particles. An example of this is PSMA-targeted radionuclide therapy with radioisotopes such as lutetium-177 (^{177}Lu), among those commonly used.

Early trials utilizing PSMA-targeted therapies have shown promising results. The TheraP trial compared PSMA-targeted therapy using ^{117}Lu-PSMA-617 to Cabazitaxel in men with metastatic castrate resistance prostate cancer (mCRPC) as a second-line treatment following docetaxel. It found an improved PSA response (66% vs. 37%) and reduced adverse effects in the ^{117}Lu-PSMA-617 arm [119]. The VISION trial also studied PSMA-targeted therapy using ^{117}Lu-PSMA-617 in men with mCRPC. Specifically, it looked at those who had ongoing disease progression despite treatment with both ADT and chemotherapy. Of note, patients who had only received one taxane therapy were ineligible if they were a candidate to receive a second. It compared patients receiving standard care alone (limited by the trial protocol to not include chemotherapy, radium-223, or immunotherapy), and those receiving PSMA-targeted therapy with ^{117}Lu-PSMA-617 in addition to standard care. It found that PSMA-targeted therapy delayed progression and improved overall survival (15.3 vs. 11.3 months) when used in addition to standard care, and that it was safe and well-tolerated [120]. At present, based on the current evidence, the EAU consensus is that its use outside of clinical trials should be limited to patients with mCRPC [121]. Where exactly it fits within the pathway of treatment for these patients remains unclear at present. However, several trials are in progress, including those examining its use prior to taxane therapy, alongside a variety of other therapies and in metastatic hormone sensitive prostate cancer (mHSPC).

The recognized limitations of this approach include the reliance on PSMA expression to effectively target. This can be quantified on diagnostic PSMA PET/CT using standardized update values (SUV) with an increased response to treatment seen in those with a higher SUV and no response in low levels [122]. As a result, PSMA lesion positivity has been used as inclusion criteria for some clinical trials, though the definition used has varied. The TheraP trial restricted inclusion to PSMA positivity with an SUVmax (the maximum standardised uptake value) of at least 20 at a site of disease and SUVmax > 10 at all other measurable metastatic disease [119]. The VISION trial required at least one PSMA-positive metastatic lesion where PSMA positivity was defined as an uptake greater than that within the liver [120]. Additionally steps were taken to exclude PSMA negative disease; TheraP patients also underwent ^{18}F-FDG PET/CT, and those with FDG positive and PSMA negative disease were excluded, whereas VISION excluded patients with PSMA uptake equal/lower than within liver in metastasis above a predefined size (>2.5 cm in lymph nodes or >1 cm in solid organs or bone lesions) [119,120]. Within VISION, 95.1% had a positive lesion, with 8.7% of patients excluded for PSMA negative lesions [120]. In TheraP, 10% of those screened were excluded for not meeting PSMA uptake criteria, and a further 18% due to discordant FDG uptake [119]. Though a standardized criteria does not exist for eligibility for PSMA targeted therapy, these are important considerations with prognostic implications, as patients who exhibit low PSMA uptake or FDG discordant lesions have been shown to have poor outcomes [123].

Alternative PSMA-targeting therapies being developed include immunotherapy. One example of this is pasotuxizumab, which binds to PSMA and to T cells resulting in the T-cell-mediated destruction of PSMA expressing cells [124]. This, and other similar therapies, are still early in their stages of development [124,125].

7. Conclusions

The field of prostate cancer imaging is an exciting one. There is ongoing development in areas of existing well-established applications, such as diagnosis and biopsy targeting. Perhaps more exciting still is the new areas of development, in particular, the future role of theranostics in the treatment pathway. The types of imaging modality and their role in diagnosis and treatment of prostate cancer discussed within this review are summarized in Table 2.

Table 2. Summary of Imaging modalities and their role in Prostate Cancer.

Modality	Setting				
	Diagnosis	Active Surveillance	Staging	Detection of Recurrent Disease	Theranostics
CT [a]	-	-	Current Standard	-	-
MRI [b]	Current Standard (mpMRI [c])	Current Standard (mpMRI)	Current Standard (mp/whole body MRI)	-	-
Tc99 [d] Bone scan	-	-	Current Standard	-	-
SPECT [e]	-	-	Current Standard	-	-
PSMA PET [f]/CT	Evolving Role	Evolving Role	Evolving Role	Current Standard	Evolving role (Lu^{177} targeted therapy)
PSMA PET/MRI	Evolving Role	-	-	Evolving Role	-

Current standard indicated in Green. Evolving Role indicated in Yellow. [a] Computed Tomography, [b] Magnetic Resonance Imaging, [c] Multiparametric MRI, [d] Technetium 99, [e] Single Photo Emission computed tomography, [f] Prostate Specific Membrane Antigen Position Emission Tomography.

Funding: This research received no external funding.

Conflicts of Interest: The authors declare no conflict of interest.

References

1. Astraldi, A. Diagnosis of cancer of the prostate: Biopsy by rectal route. *Urol. Cutan. Rev.* **1937**, *41*, 421–422.
2. Chen, F.K.; de Castro Abreu, A.L.; Palmer, S.L. Utility of Ultrasound in the Diagnosis, Treatment, and Follow-up of Prostate Cancer: State of the Art. *J. Nucl. Med.* **2016**, *57* (Suppl. 3), 13S–18S. [CrossRef]
3. Dahnert, W.F.; Hamper, U.M.; Eggleston, J.C.; Walsh, P.C.; Sanders, R.C. Prostatic evaluation by transrectal sonography with histopathologic correlation: The echopenic appearance of early carcinoma. *Radiology* **1986**, *158*, 97–102. [CrossRef] [PubMed]
4. Eichler, K.; Hempel, S.; Wilby, J.; Myers, L.; Bachmann, L.M.; Kleijnen, J. Diagnostic value of systematic biopsy methods in the investigation of prostate cancer: A systematic review. *J. Urol.* **2006**, *175*, 1605–1612. [CrossRef]
5. Ahmed, H.U.; El-Shater Bosaily, A.; Brown, L.C.; Gabe, R.; Kaplan, R.; Parmar, M.K.; Collaco-Moraes, Y.; Ward, K.; Hindley, R.G.; Freeman, A.; et al. Diagnostic accuracy of multi-parametric MRI and TRUS biopsy in prostate cancer (PROMIS): A paired validating confirmatory study. *Lancet* **2017**, *389*, 815–822. [CrossRef]
6. Mottet, N.; van den Bergh, R.C.N.; Briers, E.; Van den Broeck, T.; Cumberbatch, M.G.; De Santis, M.; Fanti, S.; Fossati, N.; Gandaglia, G.; Gillessen, S.; et al. EAU-EANM-ESTRO-ESUR-SIOG Guidelines on Prostate Cancer-2020 Update. Part 1: Screening, Diagnosis, and Local Treatment with Curative Intent. *Eur. Urol.* **2021**, *79*, 243–262. [CrossRef] [PubMed]

7. Turkbey, B.; Rosenkrantz, A.B.; Haider, M.A.; Padhani, A.R.; Villeirs, G.; Macura, K.J.; Tempany, C.M.; Choyke, P.L.; Cornud, F.; Margolis, D.J.; et al. Prostate Imaging Reporting and Data System Version 2.1: 2019 Update of Prostate Imaging Reporting and Data System Version 2. *Eur. Urol.* **2019**, *76*, 340–351. [CrossRef]
8. Desai, S.; Costa, D.N. PI-RADS and Likert scales for structured reporting in multiparametric MR imaging of the prostate. *Br. J. Radiol.* **2022**, *95*, 20210758. [CrossRef] [PubMed]
9. Pesapane, F.; Acquasanta, M.; Meo, R.D.; Agazzi, G.M.; Tantrige, P.; Codari, M.; Schiaffino, S.; Patella, F.; Esseridou, A.; Sardanelli, F. Comparison of Sensitivity and Specificity of Biparametric versus Multiparametric Prostate MRI in the Detection of Prostate Cancer in 431 Men with Elevated Prostate-Specific Antigen Levels. *Diagnostics* **2021**, *11*, 1223. [CrossRef]
10. Russo, F.; Mazzetti, S.; Regge, D.; Ambrosini, I.; Giannini, V.; Manfredi, M.; De Luca, S.; Bollito, E.; Porpiglia, F. Diagnostic Accuracy of Single-plane Biparametric and Multiparametric Magnetic Resonance Imaging in Prostate Cancer: A Randomized Noninferiority Trial in Biopsy-naive Men. *Eur. Urol. Oncol.* **2021**, *4*, 855–862. [CrossRef]
11. Kang, Z.; Min, X.; Weinreb, J.; Li, Q.; Feng, Z.; Wang, L. Abbreviated Biparametric Versus Standard Multiparametric MRI for Diagnosis of Prostate Cancer: A Systematic Review and Meta-Analysis. *AJR Am. J. Roentgenol.* **2019**, *212*, 357–365. [CrossRef] [PubMed]
12. Woo, S.; Suh, C.H.; Kim, S.Y.; Cho, J.Y.; Kim, S.H.; Moon, M.H. Head-to-Head Comparison Between Biparametric and Multiparametric MRI for the Diagnosis of Prostate Cancer: A Systematic Review and Meta-Analysis. *AJR Am. J. Roentgenol.* **2018**, *211*, W226–W241. [CrossRef] [PubMed]
13. Martin, R.M.; Donovan, J.L.; Turner, E.L.; Metcalfe, C.; Young, G.J.; Walsh, E.I.; Lane, J.A.; Noble, S.; Oliver, S.E.; Evans, S.; et al. Effect of a Low-Intensity PSA-Based Screening Intervention on Prostate Cancer Mortality: The CAP Randomized Clinical Trial. *JAMA* **2018**, *319*, 883–895. [CrossRef] [PubMed]
14. Hugosson, J.; Roobol, M.J.; Mansson, M.; Tammela, T.L.J.; Zappa, M.; Nelen, V.; Kwiatkowski, M.; Lujan, M.; Carlsson, S.V.; Talala, K.M.; et al. A 16-yr Follow-up of the European Randomized study of Screening for Prostate Cancer. *Eur. Urol.* **2019**, *76*, 43–51. [CrossRef]
15. Eldred-Evans, D.; Ahmed, H.U. Population-Based Prostate Cancer Screening with Magnetic Resonance Imaging or Ultrasonography-The IP1-PROSTAGRAM Study-Reply. *JAMA Oncol.* **2021**, *7*, 1575–1576. [CrossRef]
16. Marsden, T.; Lomas, D.J.; McCartan, N.; Hadley, J.; Tuck, S.; Brown, L.; Haire, A.; Moss, C.L.; Green, S.; Van Hemelrijck, M.; et al. ReIMAGINE Prostate Cancer Screening Study: Protocol for a single-centre feasibility study inviting men for prostate cancer screening using MRI. *BMJ Open* **2021**, *11*, e048144. [CrossRef]
17. Sunnybrook Health Sciences Centre. MRI Versus PSA in Prostate Cancer Screening 2020 Updated June. Available online: https://ClinicalTrials.gov/show/NCT02799303 (accessed on 20 November 2022).
18. Tamhankar, A.S.; El-Taji, O.; Vasdev, N.; Foley, C.; Popert, R.; Adshead, J. The clinical and financial implications of a decade of prostate biopsies in the NHS: Analysis of Hospital Episode Statistics data 2008–2019. *BJU Int.* **2020**, *126*, 133–141. [CrossRef]
19. Pilatz, A.; Dimitropoulos, K.; Veeratterapillay, R.; Yuan, Y.; Omar, M.I.; MacLennan, S.; Cai, T.; Bruyere, F.; Bartoletti, R.; Koves, B.; et al. Antibiotic Prophylaxis for the Prevention of Infectious Complications following Prostate Biopsy: A Systematic Review and Meta-Analysis. *J. Urol.* **2020**, *204*, 224–230. [CrossRef]
20. Castellani, D.; Pirola, G.M.; Law, Y.X.T.; Gubbiotti, M.; Giulioni, C.; Scarcella, S.; Wroclawski, M.L.; Chan, E.; Chiu, P.K.; Teoh, J.Y.; et al. Infection Rate after Transperineal Prostate Biopsy with and without Prophylactic Antibiotics: Results from a Systematic Review and Meta-Analysis of Comparative Studies. *J. Urol.* **2022**, *207*, 25–34. [CrossRef]
21. Basourakos, S.P.; Alshak, M.N.; Lewicki, P.J.; Cheng, E.; Tzeng, M.; DeRosa, A.P.; Allaway, M.J.; Ross, A.E.; Schaeffer, E.M.; Patel, H.D.; et al. Role of Prophylactic Antibiotics in Transperineal Prostate Biopsy: A Systematic Review and Meta-analysis. *Eur. Urol. Open Sci.* **2022**, *37*, 53–63. [CrossRef]
22. Jacewicz, M.; Günzel, K.; Rud, E.; Sandbæk, G.; Magheli, A.; Busch, J.; Hinz, S.; Baco, E. Antibiotic prophylaxis versus no antibiotic prophylaxis in transperineal prostate biopsies (NORAPP): A randomised, open-label, non-inferiority trial. *Lancet Infect. Dis.* **2022**, *22*, 1465–1471. [CrossRef]
23. University of Oxford; National Institute for Health Research UK. The TRANSLATE Trial 2022 Updated December 31. Available online: https://ClinicalTrials.gov/show/NCT05179694 (accessed on 20 November 2022).
24. Kasivisvanathan, V.; Rannikko, A.S.; Borghi, M.; Panebianco, V.; Mynderse, L.A.; Vaarala, M.H.; Briganti, A.; Budaus, L.; Hellawell, G.; Hindley, R.G.; et al. MRI-Targeted or Standard Biopsy for Prostate-Cancer Diagnosis. *N. Engl. J. Med.* **2018**, *378*, 1767–1777. [CrossRef] [PubMed]
25. Rouviere, O.; Puech, P.; Renard-Penna, R.; Claudon, M.; Roy, C.; Mege-Lechevallier, F.; Decaussin-Petrucci, M.; Dubreuil-Chambardel, M.; Magaud, L.; Remontet, L.; et al. Use of prostate systematic and targeted biopsy on the basis of multiparametric MRI in biopsy-naive patients (MRI-FIRST): A prospective, multicentre, paired diagnostic study. *Lancet Oncol.* **2019**, *20*, 100–109. [CrossRef] [PubMed]
26. Elkhoury, F.F.; Felker, E.R.; Kwan, L.; Sisk, A.E.; Delfin, M.; Natarajan, S.; Marks, L.S. Comparison of Targeted vs Systematic Prostate Biopsy in Men Who Are Biopsy Naive: The Prospective Assessment of Image Registration in the Diagnosis of Prostate Cancer (PAIREDCAP) Study. *JAMA Surg.* **2019**, *154*, 811–818. [CrossRef] [PubMed]

27. van der Leest, M.; Cornel, E.; Israel, B.; Hendriks, R.; Padhani, A.R.; Hoogenboom, M.; Zamecnik, P.; Bakker, D.; Setiasti, A.Y.; Veltman, J.; et al. Head-to-head Comparison of Transrectal Ultrasound-guided Prostate Biopsy Versus Multiparametric Prostate Resonance Imaging with Subsequent Magnetic Resonance-guided Biopsy in Biopsy-naive Men with Elevated Prostate-specific Antigen: A Large Prospective Multicenter Clinical Study. *Eur. Urol.* **2019**, *75*, 570–578. [CrossRef] [PubMed]
28. Patel, M.I.; Muter, S.; Vladica, P.; Gillatt, D. Robotic-assisted magnetic resonance imaging ultrasound fusion results in higher significant cancer detection compared to cognitive prostate targeting in biopsy naive men. *Transl. Androl. Urol.* **2020**, *9*, 601–608. [CrossRef]
29. Venderink, W.; de Rooij, M.; Sedelaar, J.P.M.; Huisman, H.J.; Futterer, J.J. Elastic Versus Rigid Image Registration in Magnetic Resonance Imaging-transrectal Ultrasound Fusion Prostate Biopsy: A Systematic Review and Meta-analysis. *Eur. Urol. Focus* **2018**, *4*, 219–227. [CrossRef]
30. Venderink, W.; van Luijtelaar, A.; Bomers, J.G.R.; van der Leest, M.; Hulsbergen-van de Kaa, C.; Barentsz, J.O.; Sedelaar, J.P.M.; Futterer, J.J. Results of Targeted Biopsy in Men with Magnetic Resonance Imaging Lesions Classified Equivocal, Likely or Highly Likely to Be Clinically Significant Prostate Cancer. *Eur. Urol.* **2018**, *73*, 353–360. [CrossRef]
31. Vilanova, J.C.; Perez de Tudela, A.; Puig, J.; Hoogenboom, M.; Barcelo, J.; Planas, M.; Sala, S.; Thio-Henestrosa, S. Robotic-assisted transrectal MRI-guided biopsy. Technical feasibility and role in the current diagnosis of prostate cancer: An initial single-center experience. *Abdom. Radiol.* **2020**, *45*, 4150–4159. [CrossRef]
32. Barral, M.; Lefevre, A.; Camparo, P.; Hoogenboom, M.; Pierre, T.; Soyer, P.; Cornud, F. In-Bore Transrectal MRI-Guided Biopsy with Robotic Assistance in the Diagnosis of Prostate Cancer: An Analysis of 57 Patients. *AJR Am. J. Roentgenol.* **2019**, *213*, W171–W179. [CrossRef]
33. Wegelin, O.; Exterkate, L.; van der Leest, M.; Kummer, J.A.; Vreuls, W.; de Bruin, P.C.; Bosch, J.; Barentsz, J.O.; Somford, D.M.; van Melick, H.H.E. The FUTURE Trial: A Multicenter Randomised Controlled Trial on Target Biopsy Techniques Based on Magnetic Resonance Imaging in the Diagnosis of Prostate Cancer in Patients with Prior Negative Biopsies. *Eur. Urol.* **2019**, *75*, 582–590. [CrossRef]
34. Bass, E.J.; Pantovic, A.; Connor, M.J.; Loeb, S.; Rastinehad, A.R.; Winkler, M.; Gabe, R.; Ahmed, H.U. Diagnostic accuracy of magnetic resonance imaging targeted biopsy techniques compared to transrectal ultrasound guided biopsy of the prostate: A systematic review and meta-analysis. *Prostate Cancer Prostatic Dis.* **2021**, *25*, 174–179. [CrossRef] [PubMed]
35. Costa, D.N.; Goldberg, K.; Leon, A.D.; Lotan, Y.; Xi, Y.; Aziz, M.; Freifeld, Y.; Margulis, V.; Raj, G.; Roehrborn, C.G.; et al. Magnetic Resonance Imaging-guided In-bore and Magnetic Resonance Imaging-transrectal Ultrasound Fusion Targeted Prostate Biopsies: An Adjusted Comparison of Clinically Significant Prostate Cancer Detection Rate. *Eur. Urol. Oncol.* **2019**, *2*, 397–404. [CrossRef] [PubMed]
36. Del Monte, M.; Cipollari, S.; Del Giudice, F.; Pecoraro, M.; Bicchetti, M.; Messina, E.; Dehghanpour, A.; Ciardi, A.; Sciarra, A.; Catalano, C.; et al. MRI-directed biopsy for primary detection of prostate cancer in a population of 223 men: MRI In-Bore vs MRI-transrectal ultrasound fusion-targeted techniques. *Br. J. Radiol.* **2022**, *95*, 20210528. [CrossRef]
37. Crisan, G.; Moldovean-Cioroianu, N.S.; Timaru, D.G.; Andries, G.; Cainap, C.; Chis, V. Radiopharmaceuticals for PET and SPECT Imaging: A Literature Review over the Last Decade. *Int. J. Mol. Sci.* **2022**, *23*, 5023. [CrossRef]
38. Watakabe, T.; Toya, R.; Saito, T.; Matsuyama, T.; Shiraishi, S.; Kai, Y.; Shimohigashi, Y.; Oya, N. High Spatial Resolution Digital Positron Emission Tomography Images with Dedicated Source-to-background Algorithm for Radiotherapy Planning. *Anticancer Res.* **2020**, *40*, 2567–2572. [CrossRef] [PubMed]
39. Farsad, M.; Schiavina, R.; Castellucci, P.; Nanni, C.; Corti, B.; Martorana, G.; Canini, R.; Grigioni, W.; Boschi, S.; Marengo, M.; et al. Detection and localization of prostate cancer: Correlation of (11)C-choline PET/CT with histopathologic step-section analysis. *J. Nucl. Med.* **2005**, *46*, 1642–1649.
40. Souvatzoglou, M.; Weirich, G.; Schwarzenboeck, S.; Maurer, T.; Schuster, T.; Bundschuh, R.A.; Eiber, M.; Herrmann, K.; Kuebler, H.; Wester, H.J.; et al. The sensitivity of [11C]choline PET/CT to localize prostate cancer depends on the tumor configuration. *Clin. Cancer Res.* **2011**, *17*, 3751–3759. [CrossRef]
41. Murphy, G.P.; Elgamal, A.A.; Su, S.L.; Bostwick, D.G.; Holmes, E.H. Current evaluation of the tissue localization and diagnostic utility of prostate specific membrane antigen. *Cancer* **1998**, *83*, 2259–2269. [CrossRef]
42. Perner, S.; Hofer, M.D.; Kim, R.; Shah, R.B.; Li, H.; Moller, P.; Hautmann, R.E.; Gschwend, J.E.; Kuefer, R.; Rubin, M.A. Prostate-specific membrane antigen expression as a predictor of prostate cancer progression. *Hum. Pathol.* **2007**, *38*, 696–701. [CrossRef]
43. Salas Fragomeni, R.A.; Amir, T.; Sheikhbahaei, S.; Harvey, S.C.; Javadi, M.S.; Solnes, L.B.; Kiess, A.P.; Allaf, M.E.; Pomper, M.G.; Gorin, M.A.; et al. Imaging of Nonprostate Cancers Using PSMA-Targeted Radiotracers: Rationale, Current State of the Field, and a Call to Arms. *J. Nucl. Med.* **2018**, *59*, 871–877. [CrossRef] [PubMed]
44. Sheikhbahaei, S.; Afshar-Oromieh, A.; Eiber, M.; Solnes, L.B.; Javadi, M.S.; Ross, A.E.; Pienta, K.J.; Allaf, M.E.; Haberkorn, U.; Pomper, M.G.; et al. Pearls and pitfalls in clinical interpretation of prostate-specific membrane antigen (PSMA)-targeted PET imaging. *Eur. J. Nucl. Med. Mol. Imaging* **2017**, *44*, 2117–2136. [CrossRef] [PubMed]
45. Afshar-Oromieh, A.; Malcher, A.; Eder, M.; Eisenhut, M.; Linhart, H.G.; Hadaschik, B.A.; Holland-Letz, T.; Giesel, F.L.; Kratochwil, C.; Haufe, S.; et al. PET imaging with a [68Ga]gallium-labelled PSMA ligand for the diagnosis of prostate cancer: Biodistribution in humans and first evaluation of tumour lesions. *Eur. J. Nucl. Med. Mol. Imaging* **2013**, *40*, 486–495. [CrossRef]

46. Afshar-Oromieh, A.; Debus, N.; Uhrig, M.; Hope, T.A.; Evans, M.J.; Holland-Letz, T.; Giesel, F.L.; Kopka, K.; Hadaschik, B.; Kratochwil, C.; et al. Impact of long-term androgen deprivation therapy on PSMA ligand PET/CT in patients with castration-sensitive prostate cancer. *Eur. J. Nucl. Med. Mol. Imaging* **2018**, *45*, 2045–2054. [CrossRef]
47. Ettala, O.; Malaspina, S.; Tuokkola, T.; Luoto, P.; Loyttyniemi, E.; Bostrom, P.J.; Kemppainen, J. Prospective study on the effect of short-term androgen deprivation therapy on PSMA uptake evaluated with (68)Ga-PSMA-11 PET/MRI in men with treatment-naive prostate cancer. *Eur. J. Nucl. Med. Mol. Imaging* **2020**, *47*, 665–673. [CrossRef] [PubMed]
48. Malaspina, S.; Ettala, O.; Tolvanen, T.; Rajander, J.; Eskola, O.; Bostrom, P.J.; Kemppainen, J. Flare on [(18)F]PSMA-1007 PET/CT after short-term androgen deprivation therapy and its correlation to FDG uptake: Possible marker of tumor aggressiveness in treatment-naive metastatic prostate cancer patients. *Eur. J. Nucl. Med. Mol. Imaging* **2022**, *50*, 613–621. [CrossRef]
49. Onal, C.; Guler, O.C.; Torun, N.; Reyhan, M.; Yapar, A.F. The effect of androgen deprivation therapy on (68)Ga-PSMA tracer uptake in non-metastatic prostate cancer patients. *Eur. J. Nucl. Med. Mol. Imaging* **2020**, *47*, 632–641. [CrossRef]
50. Tseng, J.R.; Chang, S.H.; Wu, Y.Y.; Fan, K.H.; Yu, K.J.; Yang, L.Y.; Hsiao, I.T.; Liu, F.Y.; Pang, S.T. Impact of Three-Month Androgen Deprivation Therapy on [68Ga]Ga-PSMA-11 PET/CT Indices in Men with Advanced Prostate Cancer-Results from a Pilot Prospective Study. *Cancers* **2022**, *14*, 1329. [CrossRef]
51. Eiber, M.; Weirich, G.; Holzapfel, K.; Souvatzoglou, M.; Haller, B.; Rauscher, I.; Beer, A.J.; Wester, H.J.; Gschwend, J.; Schwaiger, M.; et al. Simultaneous (68)Ga-PSMA HBED-CC PET/MRI Improves the Localization of Primary Prostate Cancer. *Eur. Urol.* **2016**, *70*, 829–836. [CrossRef]
52. Hicks, R.M.; Simko, J.P.; Westphalen, A.C.; Nguyen, H.G.; Greene, K.L.; Zhang, L.; Carroll, P.R.; Hope, T.A. Diagnostic Accuracy of (68)Ga-PSMA-11 PET/MRI Compared with Multiparametric MRI in the Detection of Prostate Cancer. *Radiology* **2018**, *289*, 730–737. [CrossRef]
53. Margel, D.; Bernstine, H.; Groshar, D.; Ber, Y.; Nezrit, O.; Segal, N.; Yakimov, M.; Baniel, J.; Domachevsky, L. Diagnostic Performance of (68)Ga Prostate-specific Membrane Antigen PET/MRI Compared with Multiparametric MRI for Detecting Clinically Significant Prostate Cancer. *Radiology* **2021**, *301*, 379–386. [CrossRef]
54. Jena, A.; Taneja, R.; Taneja, S.; Singh, A.; Kumar, V.; Agarwal, A.; Subramanian, N. Improving Diagnosis of Primary Prostate Cancer with Combined (68)Ga-Prostate-Specific Membrane Antigen-HBED-CC Simultaneous PET and Multiparametric MRI and Clinical Parameters. *AJR Am. J. Roentgenol* **2018**, *211*, 1246–1253. [CrossRef] [PubMed]
55. Scheltema, M.J.; Chang, J.I.; Stricker, P.D.; van Leeuwen, P.J.; Nguyen, Q.A.; Ho, B.; Delprado, W.; Lee, J.; Thompson, J.E.; Cusick, T.; et al. Diagnostic accuracy of (68) Ga-prostate-specific membrane antigen (PSMA) positron-emission tomography (PET) and multiparametric (mp)MRI to detect intermediate-grade intra-prostatic prostate cancer using whole-mount pathology: Impact of the addition of (68) Ga-PSMA PET to mpMRI. *BJU Int.* **2019**, *124* (Suppl. 1), 42–49. [CrossRef] [PubMed]
56. Al-Bayati, M.; Grueneisen, J.; Lutje, S.; Sawicki, L.M.; Suntharalingam, S.; Tschirdewahn, S.; Forsting, M.; Rubben, H.; Herrmann, K.; Umutlu, L.; et al. Integrated 68Gallium Labelled Prostate-Specific Membrane Antigen-11 Positron Emission Tomography/Magnetic Resonance Imaging Enhances Discriminatory Power of Multi-Parametric Prostate Magnetic Resonance Imaging. *Urol. Int.* **2018**, *100*, 164–171. [CrossRef]
57. Kawada, T.; Yanagisawa, T.; Rajwa, P.; Sari Motlagh, R.; Mostafaei, H.; Quhal, F.; Laukhtina, E.; Aydh, A.; Konig, F.; Pallauf, M.; et al. Diagnostic Performance of Prostate-specific Membrane Antigen Positron Emission Tomography-targeted biopsy for Detection of Clinically Significant Prostate Cancer: A Systematic Review and Meta-analysis. *Eur. Urol. Oncol.* **2022**, *5*, 390–400. [CrossRef]
58. Emmett, L.; Buteau, J.; Papa, N.; Moon, D.; Thompson, J.; Roberts, M.J.; Rasiah, K.; Pattison, D.A.; Yaxley, J.; Thomas, P.; et al. The Additive Diagnostic Value of Prostate-specific Membrane Antigen Positron Emission Tomography Computed Tomography to Multiparametric Magnetic Resonance Imaging Triage in the Diagnosis of Prostate Cancer (PRIMARY): A Prospective Multicentre Study. *Eur. Urol.* **2021**, *80*, 682–689. [CrossRef] [PubMed]
59. Peter MacCallum Cancer Centre, Australia; St Vincent's Hospital, Sydney. PSMA PET Additive Value for Prostate Cancer Diagnosis in Men with Negative/Equivocal MRI. Available online: https://ClinicalTrials.gov/show/NCT05154162:2022 (accessed on 20 November 2022).
60. Patel, H.D.; Johnson, M.H.; Pierorazio, P.M.; Sozio, S.M.; Sharma, R.; Iyoha, E.; Bass, E.B.; Allaf, M.E. Diagnostic Accuracy and Risks of Biopsy in the Diagnosis of a Renal Mass Suspicious for Localized Renal Cell Carcinoma: Systematic Review of the Literature. *J. Urol.* **2016**, *195*, 1340–1347. [CrossRef]
61. NICE. *Prostate Cancer: Diagnosis and Management [NG131]*; National Institute for Health and Care Excellence: London, UK, 2021.
62. Carlsson, S.; Benfante, N.; Alvim, R.; Sjoberg, D.D.; Vickers, A.; Reuter, V.E.; Fine, S.W.; Vargas, H.A.; Wiseman, M.; Mamoor, M.; et al. Long-Term Outcomes of Active Surveillance for Prostate Cancer: The Memorial Sloan Kettering Cancer Center Experience. *J. Urol.* **2020**, *203*, 1122–1127. [CrossRef] [PubMed]
63. Klotz, L.; Vesprini, D.; Sethukavalan, P.; Jethava, V.; Zhang, L.; Jain, S.; Yamamoto, T.; Mamedov, A.; Loblaw, A. Long-term follow-up of a large active surveillance cohort of patients with prostate cancer. *J. Clin. Oncol.* **2015**, *33*, 272–277. [CrossRef] [PubMed]
64. Moore, C.M.; Giganti, F.; Albertsen, P.; Allen, C.; Bangma, C.; Briganti, A.; Carroll, P.; Haider, M.; Kasivisvanathan, V.; Kirkham, A.; et al. Reporting Magnetic Resonance Imaging in Men on Active Surveillance for Prostate Cancer: The PRECISE Recommendations-A Report of a European School of Oncology Task Force. *Eur. Urol.* **2017**, *71*, 648–655. [CrossRef]

65. Sushentsev, N.; Rundo, L.; Blyuss, O.; Nazarenko, T.; Suvorov, A.; Gnanapragasam, V.J.; Sala, E.; Barrett, T. Comparative performance of MRI-derived PRECISE scores and delta-radiomics models for the prediction of prostate cancer progression in patients on active surveillance. *Eur. Radiol.* **2022**, *32*, 680–689. [CrossRef] [PubMed]
66. Hettiarachchi, D.; Geraghty, R.; Rice, P.; Sachdeva, A.; Nambiar, A.; Johnson, M.; Gujadhur, R.; McNeill, M.; Haslam, P.; Soomro, N.; et al. Can the Use of Serial Multiparametric Magnetic Resonance Imaging During Active Surveillance of Prostate Cancer Avoid the Need for Prostate Biopsies?-A Systematic Diagnostic Test Accuracy Review. *Eur. Urol. Oncol.* **2021**, *4*, 426–436. [CrossRef] [PubMed]
67. Rajwa, P.; Pradere, B.; Quhal, F.; Mori, K.; Laukhtina, E.; Huebner, N.A.; D'Andrea, D.; Krzywon, A.; Shim, S.R.; Baltzer, P.A.; et al. Reliability of Serial Prostate Magnetic Resonance Imaging to Detect Prostate Cancer Progression During Active Surveillance: A Systematic Review and Meta-analysis. *Eur. Urol.* **2021**, *80*, 549–563. [CrossRef] [PubMed]
68. Luiting, H.B.; Remmers, S.; Boeve, E.R.; Valdagni, R.; Chiu, P.K.; Semjonow, A.; Berge, V.; Tully, K.H.; Rannikko, A.S.; Staerman, F.; et al. A Multivariable Approach Using Magnetic Resonance Imaging to Avoid a Protocol-based Prostate Biopsy in Men on Active Surveillance for Prostate Cancer-Data from the International Multicenter Prospective PRIAS Study. *Eur. Urol. Oncol.* **2022**, *5*, 651–658. [CrossRef]
69. Pepe, P.; Roscigno, M.; Pepe, L.; Panella, P.; Tamburo, M.; Marletta, G.; Savoca, F.; Candiano, G.; Cosentino, S.; Ippolito, M.; et al. Could 68Ga-PSMA PET/CT Evaluation Reduce the Number of Scheduled Prostate Biopsies in Men Enrolled in Active Surveillance Protocols? *J. Clin. Med.* **2022**, *11*, 3473. [CrossRef]
70. de Rooij, M.; Hamoen, E.H.; Witjes, J.A.; Barentsz, J.O.; Rovers, M.M. Accuracy of Magnetic Resonance Imaging for Local Staging of Prostate Cancer: A Diagnostic Meta-analysis. *Eur. Urol.* **2016**, *70*, 233–245. [CrossRef]
71. Zhang, F.; Liu, C.L.; Chen, Q.; Shao, S.C.; Chen, S.Q. Accuracy of multiparametric magnetic resonance imaging for detecting extracapsular extension in prostate cancer: A systematic review and meta-analysis. *Br. J. Radiol.* **2019**, *92*, 20190480. [CrossRef]
72. Gandaglia, G.; Ploussard, G.; Valerio, M.; Marra, G.; Moschini, M.; Martini, A.; Roumiguie, M.; Fossati, N.; Stabile, A.; Beauval, J.B.; et al. Prognostic Implications of Multiparametric Magnetic Resonance Imaging and Concomitant Systematic Biopsy in Predicting Biochemical Recurrence after Radical Prostatectomy in Prostate Cancer Patients Diagnosed with Magnetic Resonance Imaging-targeted Biopsy. *Eur. Urol. Oncol.* **2020**, *3*, 739–747. [CrossRef]
73. Sandeman, K.; Eineluoto, J.T.; Pohjonen, J.; Erickson, A.; Kilpelainen, T.P.; Jarvinen, P.; Santti, H.; Petas, A.; Matikainen, M.; Marjasuo, S.; et al. Prostate MRI added to CAPRA, MSKCC and Partin cancer nomograms significantly enhances the prediction of adverse findings and biochemical recurrence after radical prostatectomy. *PLoS ONE* **2020**, *15*, e0235779. [CrossRef]
74. Tan, N.; Shen, L.; Khoshnoodi, P.; Alcala, H.E.; Yu, W.; Hsu, W.; Reiter, R.E.; Lu, D.Y.; Raman, S.S. Pathological and 3 Tesla Volumetric Magnetic Resonance Imaging Predictors of Biochemical Recurrence after Robotic Assisted Radical Prostatectomy: Correlation with Whole Mount Histopathology. *J. Urol.* **2018**, *199*, 1218–1223. [CrossRef]
75. Partin, A.W.; Mangold, L.A.; Lamm, D.M.; Walsh, P.C.; Epstein, J.I.; Pearson, J.D. Contemporary update of prostate cancer staging nomograms (Partin Tables) for the new millennium. *Urology* **2001**, *58*, 843–848. [CrossRef] [PubMed]
76. Jaderling, F.; Akre, O.; Aly, M.; Bjorklund, J.; Olsson, M.; Adding, C.; Oberg, M.; Blomqvist, L.; Nyberg, T.; Wiklund, P.; et al. Preoperative staging using magnetic resonance imaging and risk of positive surgical margins after prostate-cancer surgery. *Prostate Cancer Prostatic Dis.* **2019**, *22*, 391–398. [CrossRef] [PubMed]
77. Leitsmann, C.; Uhlig, A.; Bremmer, F.; Mut, T.T.; Ahyai, S.; Reichert, M.; Leitsmann, M.; Trojan, L.; Popeneciu, I.V. Impact of mpMRI targeted biopsy on intraoperative nerve-sparing (NeuroSAFE) during robot-assisted laparoscopic radical prostatectomy. *Prostate* **2022**, *82*, 493–501. [CrossRef] [PubMed]
78. Gietelink, L.; Jansen, B.H.E.; Oprea-Lager, D.E.; Nieuwenhuijzen, J.A.; Vis, A.N. Preoperative multiparametric MRI does not lower positive surgical margin rate in a large series of patients undergoing robot-assisted radical prostatectomy. *J. Robot. Surg.* **2022**, *16*, 273–278. [CrossRef] [PubMed]
79. Hovels, A.M.; Heesakkers, R.A.; Adang, E.M.; Jager, G.J.; Strum, S.; Hoogeveen, Y.L.; Severens, J.L.; Barentsz, J.O. The diagnostic accuracy of CT and MRI in the staging of pelvic lymph nodes in patients with prostate cancer: A meta-analysis. *Clin. Radiol.* **2008**, *63*, 387–395. [CrossRef] [PubMed]
80. Van Nieuwenhove, S.; Van Damme, J.; Padhani, A.R.; Vandecaveye, V.; Tombal, B.; Wuts, J.; Pasoglou, V.; Lecouvet, F.E. Whole-body magnetic resonance imaging for prostate cancer assessment: Current status and future directions. *J. Magn. Reson. Imaging* **2022**, *55*, 653–680. [CrossRef] [PubMed]
81. Giovanella, L.; Castellani, M.; Suriano, S.; Ruberto, T.; Ceriani, L.; Tagliabue, L.; Lucignani, G. Multi-field-of-view SPECT is superior to whole-body scanning for assessing metastatic bone disease in patients with prostate cancer. *Tumori* **2011**, *97*, 629–633. [CrossRef]
82. Han, L.J.; Au-Yong, T.K.; Tong, W.C.; Chu, K.S.; Szeto, L.T.; Wong, C.P. Comparison of bone single-photon emission tomography and planar imaging in the detection of vertebral metastases in patients with back pain. *Eur. J. Nucl. Med.* **1998**, *25*, 635–638. [CrossRef]
83. Shen, G.; Deng, H.; Hu, S.; Jia, Z. Comparison of choline-PET/CT, MRI, SPECT, and bone scintigraphy in the diagnosis of bone metastases in patients with prostate cancer: A meta-analysis. *Skelet. Radiol.* **2014**, *43*, 1503–1513. [CrossRef]
84. Zhou, J.; Gou, Z.; Wu, R.; Yuan, Y.; Yu, G.; Zhao, Y. Comparison of PSMA-PET/CT, choline-PET/CT, NaF-PET/CT, MRI, and bone scintigraphy in the diagnosis of bone metastases in patients with prostate cancer: A systematic review and meta-analysis. *Skeletal. Radiol.* **2019**, *48*, 1915–1924 [CrossRef]

85. Hofman, M.S.; Lawrentschuk, N.; Francis, R.J.; Tang, C.; Vela, I.; Thomas, P.; Rutherford, N.; Martin, J.M.; Frydenberg, M.; Shakher, R.; et al. Prostate-specific membrane antigen PET-CT in patients with high-risk prostate cancer before curative-intent surgery or radiotherapy (proPSMA): A prospective, randomised, multicentre study. *Lancet* **2020**, *395*, 1208–1216. [CrossRef] [PubMed]
86. Pienta, K.J.; Gorin, M.A.; Rowe, S.P.; Carroll, P.R.; Pouliot, F.; Probst, S.; Saperstein, L.; Preston, M.A.; Alva, A.S.; Patnaik, A.; et al. A Phase 2/3 Prospective Multicenter Study of the Diagnostic Accuracy of Prostate Specific Membrane Antigen PET/CT with (18)F-DCFPyL in Prostate Cancer Patients (OSPREY). *J. Urol.* **2021**, *206*, 52–61. [CrossRef]
87. Passoni, N.M.; Fajkovic, H.; Xylinas, E.; Kluth, L.; Seitz, C.; Robinson, B.D.; Roupret, M.; Chun, F.K.; Lotan, Y.; Roehrborn, C.G.; et al. Prognosis of patients with pelvic lymph node (LN) metastasis after radical prostatectomy: Value of extranodal extension and size of the largest LN metastasis. *BJU Int.* **2014**, *114*, 503–510. [CrossRef]
88. Fossati, N.; Willemse, P.M.; Van den Broeck, T.; van den Bergh, R.C.N.; Yuan, C.Y.; Briers, E.; Bellmunt, J.; Bolla, M.; Cornford, P.; De Santis, M.; et al. The Benefits and Harms of Different Extents of Lymph Node Dissection during Radical Prostatectomy for Prostate Cancer: A Systematic Review. *Eur. Urol.* **2017**, *72*, 84–109. [CrossRef]
89. Hope, T.A.; Eiber, M.; Armstrong, W.R.; Juarez, R.; Murthy, V.; Lawhn-Heath, C.; Behr, S.C.; Zhang, L.; Barbato, F.; Ceci, F.; et al. Diagnostic Accuracy of 68Ga-PSMA-11 PET for Pelvic Nodal Metastasis Detection Prior to Radical Prostatectomy and Pelvic Lymph Node Dissection: A Multicenter Prospective Phase 3 Imaging Trial. *JAMA Oncol.* **2021**, *7*, 1635–1642. [CrossRef]
90. Brembilla, G.; Dell'Oglio, P.; Stabile, A.; Ambrosi, A.; Cristel, G.; Brunetti, L.; Damascelli, A.; Freschi, M.; Esposito, A.; Briganti, A.; et al. Preoperative multiparametric MRI of the prostate for the prediction of lymph node metastases in prostate cancer patients treated with extended pelvic lymph node dissection. *Eur. Radiol.* **2018**, *28*, 1969–1976. [CrossRef]
91. Stabile, A.; Pellegrino, A.; Mazzone, E.; Cannoletta, D.; de Angelis, M.; Barletta, F.; Scuderi, S.; Cucchiara, V.; Gandaglia, G.; Raggi, D.; et al. Can Negative Prostate-specific Membrane Antigen Positron Emission Tomography/Computed Tomography Avoid the Need for Pelvic Lymph Node Dissection in Newly Diagnosed Prostate Cancer Patients? A Systematic Review and Meta-analysis with Backup Histology as Reference Standard. *Eur. Urol. Oncol.* **2022**, *5*, 651–658. [CrossRef]
92. Gandaglia, G.; Mazzone, E.; Stabile, A.; Pellegrino, A.; Cucchiara, V.; Barletta, F.; Scuderi, S.; Robesti, D.; Leni, R.; Samanes Gajate, A.M.; et al. Prostate-specific membrane antigen Radioguided Surgery to Detect Nodal Metastases in Primary Prostate Cancer Patients Undergoing Robot-assisted Radical Prostatectomy and Extended Pelvic Lymph Node Dissection: Results of a Planned Interim Analysis of a Prospective Phase 2 Study. *Eur. Urol.* **2022**, *82*, 411–418. [CrossRef]
93. Parker, C.C.; James, N.D.; Brawley, C.D.; Clarke, N.W.; Hoyle, A.P.; Ali, A.; Ritchie, A.W.S.; Attard, G.; Chowdhury, S.; Cross, W.; et al. Radiotherapy to the primary tumour for newly diagnosed, metastatic prostate cancer (STAMPEDE): A randomised controlled phase 3 trial. *Lancet* **2018**, *392*, 2353–2366. [CrossRef]
94. Shemshaki, H.; Al-Mamari, S.A.; Geelani, I.A.; Kumar, S. Cytoreductive radical prostatectomy versus systemic therapy and radiation therapy in metastatic prostate cancer: A systematic review and meta-analysis. *Urologia* **2022**, *89*, 16–30. [CrossRef]
95. Culp, S.H.; Schellhammer, P.F.; Williams, M.B. Might men diagnosed with metastatic prostate cancer benefit from definitive treatment of the primary tumor? A SEER-based study. *Eur. Urol.* **2014**, *65*, 1058–1066. [CrossRef] [PubMed]
96. Ranasinghe, W.; Chapin, B.F.; Kim, I.Y.; Sooriakumaran, P.; Lawrentschuk, N. The cytoreductive prostatectomy in metastatic prostate cancer: What the individual trials are hoping to answer. *BJU Int.* **2020**, *125*, 792–800. [CrossRef] [PubMed]
97. Connor, M.J.; Shah, T.T.; Smigielska, K.; Day, E.; Sukumar, J.; Fiorentino, F.; Sarwar, N.; Gonzalez, M.; Falconer, A.; Klimowska-Nassar, N.; et al. Additional Treatments to the Local tumour for metastatic prostate cancer-Assessment of Novel Treatment Algorithms (IP2-ATLANTA): Protocol for a multicentre, phase II randomised controlled trial. *BMJ Open* **2021**, *11*, e042953. [CrossRef] [PubMed]
98. Ost, P.; Reynders, D.; Decaestecker, K.; Fonteyne, V.; Lumen, N.; De Bruycker, A.; Lambert, B.; Delrue, L.; Bultijnck, R.; Claeys, T.; et al. Surveillance or Metastasis-Directed Therapy for Oligometastatic Prostate Cancer Recurrence: A Prospective, Randomized, Multicenter Phase II Trial. *J. Clin. Oncol.* **2018**, *36*, 446–453. [CrossRef]
99. Artigas, C.; Diamand, R.; Shagera, Q.A.; Plouznikoff, N.; Fokoue, F.; Otte, F.X.; Gil, T.; Peltier, A.; Van Gestel, D.; Flamen, P. Oligometastatic Disease Detection with (68)Ga-PSMA-11 PET/CT in Hormone-Sensitive Prostate Cancer Patients (HSPC) with Biochemical Recurrence after Radical Prostatectomy: Predictive Factors and Clinical Impact. *Cancers* **2021**, *13*, 4982. [CrossRef] [PubMed]
100. Morawitz, J.; Kirchner, J.; Lakes, J.; Bruckmann, N.M.; Mamlins, E.; Hiester, A.; Aissa, J.; Loberg, C.; Schimmoller, L.; Arsov, C.; et al. PSMA PET/CT vs. CT alone in newly diagnosed biochemical recurrence of prostate cancer after radical prostatectomy: Comparison of detection rates and therapeutic implications. *Eur. J. Radiol.* **2021**, *136*, 109556. [CrossRef]
101. Morris, M.J.; Rowe, S.P.; Gorin, M.A.; Saperstein, L.; Pouliot, F.; Josephson, D.; Wong, J.Y.C.; Pantel, A.R.; Cho, S.Y.; Gage, K.L.; et al. Diagnostic Performance of (18)F-DCFPyL-PET/CT in Men with Biochemically Recurrent Prostate Cancer: Results from the CONDOR Phase III, Multicenter Study. *Clin. Cancer Res.* **2021**, *27*, 3674–3682. [CrossRef]
102. Wang, R.; Shen, G.; Huang, M.; Tian, R. The Diagnostic Role of (18)F-Choline, (18)F-Fluciclovine and (18)F-PSMA PET/CT in the Detection of Prostate Cancer with Biochemical Recurrence: A Meta-Analysis. *Front. Oncol.* **2021**, *11*, 684629. [CrossRef]
103. Ma, W.; Mao, J.; Yang, J.; Wang, T.; Zhao, Z.H. Comparing the diagnostic performance of radiotracers in prostate cancer biochemical recurrence: A systematic review and meta-analysis. *Eur. Radiol.* **2022**, *32*, 7374–7385. [CrossRef]

104. Tan, N.; Oyoyo, U.; Bavadian, N.; Ferguson, N.; Mukkamala, A.; Calais, J.; Davenport, M.S. PSMA-targeted Radiotracers versus (18)F Fluciclovine for the Detection of Prostate Cancer Biochemical Recurrence after Definitive Therapy: A Systematic Review and Meta-Analysis. *Radiology* **2020**, *296*, 44–55. [CrossRef]
105. Afshar-Oromieh, A.; Zechmann, C.M.; Malcher, A.; Eder, M.; Eisenhut, M.; Linhart, H.G.; Holland-Letz, T.; Hadaschik, B.A.; Giesel, F.L.; Debus, J.; et al. Comparison of PET imaging with a (68)Ga-labelled PSMA ligand and (18)F-choline-based PET/CT for the diagnosis of recurrent prostate cancer. *Eur. J. Nucl. Med. Mol. Imaging* **2014**, *41*, 11–20. [CrossRef] [PubMed]
106. Calais, J.; Ceci, F.; Eiber, M.; Hope, T.A.; Hofman, M.S.; Rischpler, C.; Bach-Gansmo, T.; Nanni, C.; Savir-Baruch, B.; Elashoff, D.; et al. (18)F-fluciclovine PET-CT and (68)Ga-PSMA-11 PET-CT in patients with early biochemical recurrence after prostatectomy: A prospective, single-centre, single-arm, comparative imaging trial. *Lancet Oncol.* **2019**, *20*, 1286–1294. [CrossRef] [PubMed]
107. Treglia, G.; Pereira Mestre, R.; Ferrari, M.; Bosetti, D.G.; Pascale, M.; Oikonomou, E.; De Dosso, S.; Jermini, F.; Prior, J.O.; Roggero, E.; et al. Radiolabelled choline versus PSMA PET/CT in prostate cancer restaging: A meta-analysis. *Am. J. Nucl. Med. Mol. Imaging* **2019**, *9*, 127–139. [PubMed]
108. Zhou, X.; Jiang, X.; Liu, L.; Wang, X.; Li, C.; Yao, Y.; Kou, Y.; Shen, J.; Shen, T.; Li, Z.; et al. Evaluation of (18)F-PSMA-1007 PET/CT in prostate cancer patients with biochemical recurrence after radical prostatectomy. *Transl. Oncol.* **2022**, *15*, 101292. [CrossRef] [PubMed]
109. von Eyben, F.E.; Picchio, M.; von Eyben, R.; Rhee, H.; Bauman, G. (68)Ga-Labeled Prostate-specific Membrane Antigen Ligand Positron Emission Tomography/Computed Tomography for Prostate Cancer: A Systematic Review and Meta-analysis. *Eur. Urol. Focus* **2018**, *4*, 686–693. [CrossRef]
110. Evangelista, L.; Maurer, T.; van der Poel, H.; Alongi, F.; Kunikowska, J.; Laudicella, R.; Fanti, S.; Hofman, M.S. [(68)Ga]Ga-PSMA Versus [(18)F]PSMA Positron Emission Tomography/Computed Tomography in the Staging of Primary and Recurrent Prostate Cancer. A Systematic Review of the Literature. *Eur. Urol. Oncol.* **2022**, *5*, 273–282. [CrossRef]
111. Manfredi, C.; Fernandez-Pascual, E.; Arcaniolo, D.; Emberton, M.; Sanchez-Salas, R.; Artigas Guix, C.; Bianco, F.; Cathcart, P.; Murphy, D.G.; Counago, F.; et al. The Role of Prostate-specific Membrane Antigen Positron Emission Tomography/Magnetic Resonance Imaging in Primary and Recurrent Prostate Cancer: A Systematic Review of the Literature. *Eur. Urol. Focus* **2022**, *8*, 942–957. [CrossRef]
112. Evangelista, L.; Zattoni, F.; Cassarino, G.; Artioli, P.; Cecchin, D.; Dal Moro, F.; Zucchetta, P. PET/MRI in prostate cancer: A systematic review and meta-analysis. *Eur. J. Nucl. Med. Mol. Imaging* **2021**, *48*, 859–873. [CrossRef]
113. Phillips, R.; Shi, W.Y.; Deek, M.; Radwan, N.; Lim, S.J.; Antonarakis, E.S.; Rowe, S.P.; Ross, A.E.; Gorin, M.A.; Deville, C.; et al. Outcomes of Observation vs Stereotactic Ablative Radiation for Oligometastatic Prostate Cancer: The ORIOLE Phase 2 Randomized Clinical Trial. *JAMA Oncol.* **2020**, *6*, 650–659. [CrossRef]
114. Deek, M.P.; Van der Eecken, K.; Sutera, P.; Deek, R.A.; Fonteyne, V.; Mendes, A.A.; Decaestecker, K.; Kiess, A.P.; Lumen, N.; Phillips, R.; et al. Long-Term Outcomes and Genetic Predictors of Response to Metastasis-Directed Therapy Versus Observation in Oligometastatic Prostate Cancer: Analysis of STOMP and ORIOLE Trials. *J. Clin. Oncol.* **2022**, *40*, 3377–3382. [CrossRef]
115. Janssen, J.; Staal, F.H.E.; Brouwer, C.L.; Langendijk, J.A.; de Jong, I.J.; van Moorselaar, R.J.A.; Schuit, E.; Verzijlbergen, J.F.; Smeenk, R.J.; Aluwini, S. Androgen Deprivation therapy for Oligo-recurrent Prostate cancer in addition to radioTherapy (ADOPT): Study protocol for a randomised phase III trial. *BMC Cancer* **2022**, *22*, 482. [CrossRef] [PubMed]
116. De Bruycker, A.; Spiessens, A.; Dirix, P.; Koutsouvelis, N.; Semac, I.; Liefhooghe, N.; Gomez-Iturriaga, A.; Everaerts, W.; Otte, F.; Papachristofilou, A.; et al. PEACE V—Salvage Treatment of OligoRecurrent nodal prostate cancer Metastases (STORM): A study protocol for a randomized controlled phase II trial. *BMC Cancer* **2020**, *20*, 406. [CrossRef]
117. Institut Cancerologie de l'Ouest; AstraZeneca. Prostate Cancer with OligometaSTatic Relapse: Combining Stereotactic Ablative Radiotherapy and Durvalumab (MEDI4736). Available online: https://ClinicalTrials.gov/show/NCT03795207:2019 (accessed on 20 November 2022).
118. Wiesing, U. Theranostics: Is it really a revolution? Evaluating a new term in medicine. *Med. Health Care Philos.* **2019**, *22*, 593–597. [CrossRef] [PubMed]
119. Hofman, M.S.; Emmett, L.; Sandhu, S.; Iravani, A.; Joshua, A.M.; Goh, J.C.; Pattison, D.A.; Tan, T.H.; Kirkwood, I.D.; Ng, S.; et al. [(177)Lu]Lu-PSMA-617 versus cabazitaxel in patients with metastatic castration-resistant prostate cancer (TheraP): A randomised, open-label, phase 2 trial. *Lancet* **2021**, *397*, 797–804. [CrossRef]
120. Sartor, O.; de Bono, J.; Chi, K.N.; Fizazi, K.; Herrmann, K.; Rahbar, K.; Tagawa, S.T.; Nordquist, L.T.; Vaishampayan, N.; El-Haddad, G.; et al. Lutetium-177-PSMA-617 for Metastatic Castration-Resistant Prostate Cancer. *N. Engl. J. Med.* **2021**, *385*, 1091–1103. [CrossRef]
121. Fanti, S.; Briganti, A.; Emmett, L.; Fizazi, K.; Gillessen, S.; Goffin, K.; Hadaschik, B.A.; Herrmann, K.; Kunikowska, J.; Maurer, T.; et al. EAU-EANM Consensus Statements on the Role of Prostate-specific Membrane Antigen Positron Emission Tomography/Computed Tomography in Patients with Prostate Cancer and with Respect to [(177)Lu]Lu-PSMA Radioligand Therapy. *Eur. Urol. Oncol.* **2022**, *5*, 530–536. [CrossRef]
122. Emmett, L.; Crumbaker, M.; Ho, B.; Willowson, K.; Eu, P.; Ratnayake, L.; Joshua, A.M.; Emmett, L.; Crumbaker, M.; Ho, B.; et al. Results of a Prospective Phase 2 Pilot Trial of (177)Lu-PSMA-617 Therapy for Metastatic Castration-Resistant Prostate Cancer Including Imaging Predictors of Treatment Response and Patterns of Progression. *Clin. Genitourin. Cancer* **2019**, *17*, 15–22. [CrossRef]

123. Thang, S.P.; Violet, J.; Sandhu, S.; Iravani, A.; Akhurst, T.; Kong, G.; Ravi Kumar, A.; Murphy, D.G.; Williams, S.G.; Hicks, R.J.; et al. Poor Outcomes for Patients with Metastatic Castration-resistant Prostate Cancer with Low Prostate-specific Membrane Antigen (PSMA) Expression Deemed Ineligible for (177)Lu-labelled PSMA Radioligand Therapy. *Eur. Urol. Oncol.* **2019**, *2*, 670–676. [CrossRef]
124. Hummel, H.D.; Kufer, P.; Grullich, C.; Seggewiss-Bernhardt, R.; Deschler-Baier, B.; Chatterjee, M.; Goebeler, M.E.; Miller, K.; de Santis, M.; Loidl, W.; et al. Pasotuxizumab, a BiTE((R)) immune therapy for castration-resistant prostate cancer: Phase I, dose-escalation study findings. *Immunotherapy* **2021**, *13*, 125–141. [CrossRef]
125. Deegen, P.; Thomas, O.; Nolan-Stevaux, O.; Li, S.; Wahl, J.; Bogner, P.; Aeffner, F.; Friedrich, M.; Liao, M.Z.; Matthes, K.; et al. The PSMA-targeting Half-life Extended BiTE Therapy AMG 160 has Potent Antitumor Activity in Preclinical Models of Metastatic Castration-resistant Prostate Cancer. *Clin. Cancer Res.* **2021**, *27*, 2928–2937. [CrossRef]

Journal of
Clinical Medicine

MDPI

Article

Determination of Whether Apex or Non-Apex Prostate Cancer Is the Best Candidate for the Use of Prostate-Specific Antigen Density to Predict Pathological Grade Group Upgrading and Upstaging after Radical Prostatectomy

Cong Huang [1,2], Shiming He [1,2], Qun He [1,2], Yanqing Gong [1,2], Gang Song [1,2,*] and Liqun Zhou [1,2,*]

1 Department of Urology, Peking University First Hospital, Beijing 100034, China
2 Institute of Urology, Peking University, National Urological Cancer Center of China, Beijing 100034, China
* Correspondence: sgbmupaper@163.com (G.S.); zhoulqmail@sina.com (L.Z.)

Abstract: Objective: Previous studies have demonstrated that prostate-specific antigen density (PSAD) may aid in predicting Gleason grade group (GG) upgrading and pathological upstaging in patients with prostate cancer (PCa). However, the differences and associations between patients with apex prostate cancer (APCa) and non-apex prostate cancer (NAPCa) have not been described. The aim of this study was to explore the different roles of PSAD in predicting GG upgrading and pathological upstaging between APCa and NAPCa. **Patients and Methods:** Five hundred and thirty-five patients who underwent prostate biopsy followed by radical prostatectomy (RP) were enrolled. All patients were diagnosed with PCa and classified as either APCa or NAPCa. Clinical and pathological variables were collected. Univariate, multivariate, and receiver operating characteristic (ROC) analyses were performed. **Results:** Of the entire cohort, 245 patients (45.8%) had GG upgrading. Multivariate analysis revealed that only PSAD (odds ratio [OR]: 4.149, $p < 0.001$) was an independent, significant predictor of upgrading. A total of 262 patients (49.0%) had pathological upstaging. Both PSAD (OR: 4.750, $p < 0.001$) and percentage of positive cores (OR: 5.108, $p = 0.002$) were independently significant predictors of upstaging. Of the 374 patients with NAPCa, 168 (44.9%) displayed GG upgrading. Multivariate analysis also showed PSAD (OR: 8.176, $p < 0.001$) was an independent predictor of upgrading. Upstaging occurred in 159 (42.5%) patients with NAPCa, and PSAD (OR: 4.973, $p < 0.001$) and percentage of positive cores (OR: 3.994, $p = 0.034$) were independently predictive of pathological upstaging. Conversely, of the 161 patients with APCa, 77 (47.8%) were identified with GG upgrading, and 103 (64.0%) patients with pathological upstaging. Multivariate analysis demonstrated that there were no significant predictors, including PSAD, for predicting GG upgrading ($p = 0.462$) and pathological upstaging ($p = 0.100$). **Conclusions:** PSAD may aid in the prediction of GG upgrading and pathological upstaging in patients with PCa. However, this may only be practical in patients with NAPCa but not with APCa. Additional biopsy cores taken from the prostatic apex region may help improve the accuracy of PSAD in predicting GG upgrading and pathological upstaging after RP.

Keywords: prostate cancer; prostate-specific antigen density; apex tumor; Gleason grade group; upgrading; upstaging

1. Introduction

Prostate cancer (PCa) is one of the mostly frequently diagnosed solid malignant tumors in men worldwide [1–3]. The treatment options for PCa are generally based upon risk stratification derived from biopsy Gleason score (GS), prostate-specific antigen (PSA), and clinical stage [4]. Thus, biopsy GS and clinical stage are principal factors in the initial assessment of patients with PCa and can inform different therapeutic strategies. Unfortunately, preoperative GS and clinical stage are often inconsistent with final pathological results after radical prostatectomy (RP). Indeed, approximately 30% to 50% of patients experience either GS upgrading or pathological upstaging after analysis of RP specimens [5]. Recently, Epstein et al. proposed an alternative, simplified PCa grading system which is based on the 2005 International Society of Urologic Pathology (ISUP) modified Gleason grading system [6]. This new Gleason grade group (GG) system, which uses the biochemical recurrence of PCa after treatment as a surrogate endpoint to define aggressive disease, appears to improve risk stratification and, consequently, clinical decision making. This grading group system was accepted by the World Health Organization (WHO) for the 2016 edition and has been validated in previous studies [7,8].

Currently, transrectal ultrasound (TRUS)-guided prostate biopsy for clinically suspected PCa detection is the standard of care. However, TRUS-guided biopsy schemes predominantly target the posterior and lateral peripheral regions of the prostate, and therefore it is difficult to sample tumors located in the prostatic anterior apex. Additionally, previous studies found that tumors primarily occurred in the anterior half of the gland at the apex to mid prostate. Both may lead to a higher false-negative rate of transrectal biopsy and increase the risk of GG upgrading and pathological upstaging [9].

The prostate-specific antigen density (PSAD) has been demonstrated to be associated with adverse pathological characteristics and poor prognosis [10,11]. Nonetheless, conflicting results were reported when assessing its ability to predict pathological upgrading and upstaging [12,13]. The controversial results may be due to various confounding factors such as biopsy scheme, tumor volume, or tumor location. To our knowledge, no study has yet compared the accuracy of PSAD in predicting upgrading and upstaging between patients with or without anteriorly apical prostate cancer (APCa).

Thus, the aim of this study was to evaluate the different performance of PSAD as a predictor of prognostic GG upgrading and pathological upstaging between APCa and non-apical prostate cancer (NAPCa).

2. Patients and Methods

2.1. Patient Selection

The institutional review board approved this retrospective study, and the requirement for informed consent was waived. Between January 2001 and April 2018, the medical records of patients who had received TRUS-guided biopsy resulting in a diagnosis of organ localized PCa (≤T2c) and underwent open, laparoscopic, or robot-assisted RP in our institution within 3 months of diagnosis were retrospectively evaluated. All patients underwent TRUS-guided systematic 12- or 13-core prostate biopsies, with the addition of at least two targeted biopsies at any area suspected of malignancy by ultrasonography. Those who received neoadjuvant androgen deprivation therapy or drugs to alter PSA values were excluded from the study. Patients with incomplete data were also excluded. Ultimately, a total of 535 patients were enrolled in the study.

All RP surgical specimens were fixed in formalin buffer (4%) after the outer surface. Specimens were sliced with standardized multiple transverse cuts, using a modified handling technique described previously by the ISUP Consensus Conference [14]. Notably, the prostatic apex (PA) of RP specimens underwent parasagittal separation and was split into two distal apical 5 mm sections. The patients were classified as either APCa or NAPCa according to the histological examination. APCa was defined as any malignant findings in the PA section, without regard to other locations.

2.2. Data Collection

Clinical and pathological data were collected from all the patients. The clinical data included age, body mass index (BMI), serum prostate-specific antigen (PSA), digital rectal examination (DRE), prostate volume (PV) evaluation via TRUS, and clinical T stage (assessed by the 2017 American Joint Committee on Cancer staging system). PSAD was calculated by dividing serum PSA by PV. The pathological data included biopsy and RP specimen GG, number of biopsy cores, number of positive cores, percentage of tumor involvement of each biopsy core, pathological T stage, extracapsular extension, seminal vesicle invasion, positive surgical margin, and lymph node invasion.

Analyses of all needle biopsies and RP specimens were centralized and performed by two dedicated genitourinary pathologists. The overall biopsy GS was based on the core with the highest GS. The overall GS of RP specimens with multifocal lesions was similarly based on the nodule with the highest GS. Gleason grading of prostatic carcinoma followed the 2005 ISUP consensus conference and was adapted to the new Gleason GG system [6]. Upgrading was regarded as an increase from one prognosis GG to another. Upstaging was defined as the pathological diagnosis of non-organ localized disease which was not clinically suspected before RP.

2.3. Statistical Analysis

Quantitative variables were described as means ± standard deviation (SD) or medians with their respective interquartile range (IQR), and differences between groups were analyzed using Student's t test or the Mann–Whitney U test, as appropriate. Qualitative variables were presented as frequencies and percentages, and differences were compared using chi-square tests. Univariate and multivariate logistic regression analyses were performed to evaluate the independent, significant variables in the prediction of GG upgrading and pathological upstaging. Receiver operating characteristic curves (ROC) were generated to assess the predictive accuracy. Statistical analyses were performed using SPSS version 20.0 (IBM Corporation, Armonk, NY, USA and MedCalc version 18.11 (MedCalc Software, Mariakerke, Belgium). All tests were two-sided and a $p < 0.05$ was considered statistically significant.

3. Results

3.1. Baseline Characteristics

The baseline clinical and pathological characteristics of the study cohort are shown in Table 1. The median age was 67 years (IQR: 62–71); the median PSA value was 10.93 ng/mL (IQR: 7.49–17.16); the median PV was 39.1 mL (IQR: 30.0–57.0); and the median PSAD was 0.26 ng/mL^2 (IQR: 0.16–0.44). In addition, the median number of biopsy cores was 13 (IQR: 12–14).

Overall, 161 patients (30.1%) were identified as having APCa. Patients presenting with APCa showed higher preoperative PSA ($p < 0.001$), lower BMI ($p = 0.005$), and higher PSAD ($p = 0.022$). Notably, patients with APCa were more likely to harbor unfavorable clinicopathological features such as a higher percentage of positive cores ($p < 0.001$), higher max core involvement ($p < 0.001$), higher post-RP GG ($p < 0.001$), higher pathological T stage ($p < 0.001$), positive surgical margin ($p < 0.001$), and extracapsular extension ($p < 0.001$). However, there were no significant differences in age ($p = 0.590$), DRE ($p = 0.228$), PV ($p = 0.175$), number of biopsy cores ($p = 0.360$), seminal vesical invasion ($p = 0.136$), and lymph node metastasis ($p = 0.346$).

3.2. The Entire Cohort

Of the entire cohort, 245 patients (45.8%) presented with GG upgrading after RP. Patients with GG upgrading had higher serum PSA value ($p < 0.001$) and higher PSAD ($p < 0.001$) compared with those who did not display GG upgrading. No significant differences were found in age ($p = 0.205$), BMI ($p = 0.418$), PV ($p = 0.119$), number of biopsy cores ($p = 0.430$), percentage of positive cores ($p = 0.599$), and max core involvement ($p = 0.393$) (Table S1). After univariate and multivariate analysis, only PSAD (odds ratio [OR]: 4.149, $p < 0.001$) was found to be an independent, significant predictor of GG upgrading (Table 2).

Table 1. Baseline characteristics of the study cohort.

	Overall (n = 535, 100%)	NAPCa (n = 374, 69.91%)	APCa (n = 161, 30.09%)	*p* Value
Age, years				0.590
Median (IQR)	67 (62–71)	67 (62–71)	67 (61–72)	
Mean ± SD	66.13 ± 6.64	66.15 ± 6.35	66.07 ± 7.29	
BMI, kg/m^2				0.005 *
Median (IQR)	24.34 (22.68–26.22)	24.22 (22.31–26.09)	24.78 (23.31–26.78)	
Mean ± SD	24.50 ± 2.87	24.27 ± 2.88	25.04 ± 2.78	
Serum PSA, ng/mL				<0.001 *
Median (IQR)	10.93 (7.49–17.16)	10.20 (7.07–16.28)	12.17 (8.55–20.98)	
Mean ± SD	14.47 ± 12.15	13.20 ± 10.69	17.48 ± 14.64	
DRE, n (%)				0.228
Normal	429 (80.2)	305 (81.6)	124 (77.0)	
Abnormal	106 (19.8)	69 (18.4)	37 (23.0)	
Biopsy GG, n (%)				0.057
1	159 (29.7)	124 (33.2)	35 (21.7)	
2	238 (44.5)	161 (43.0)	77 (47.8)	
3	78 (14.6)	51 (13.6)	27 (16.8)	
4	60 (11.2)	38 (10.2)	22 (13.7)	
Post-RP GG, n (%)				<0.001 *
1	58 (10.8)	50 (13.4)	8 (5.0)	
2	239 (44.7)	176 (47.1)	63 (39.1)	
3	163 (30.5)	94 (25.1)	69 (42.9)	
4	41 (7.7)	32 (8.6)	9 (5.6)	
5	34 (6.3)	22 (5.9)	12 (7.5)	
Prostate volume, mL				0.175
Median (IQR)	39.10 (30.00–57.00)	39.00 (29.35–56.10)	42.00 (31.00–57.50)	
Mean ± SD	46.78 ± 25.33	46.51 ± 26.62	47.40 ± 22.10	
PSAD, ng/mL^2				0.022 *
Median (IQR)	0.26 (0.16–0.44)	0.25 (0.15–0.42)	0.29 (0.18–0.50)	
Mean ± SD	0.36 ± 0.32	0.35 ± 0.32	0.40 ± 0.33	
Number of biopsy cores				0.360
Median (IQR)	13 (12–14)	13 (12–14)	13 (12–13)	
Mean ± SD	13.24 ± 2.41	13.33 ± 2.53	13.04 ± 2.11	
Number of positive cores				<0.001 *
Median (IQR)	4 (2–6)	3 (2–6)	5 (3–7)	
Mean ± SD	4.46 ± 3.06	4.10 ± 2.91	5.27 ± 3.26	
Percent positive biopsy cores, %				<0.001 *
Median (IQR)	30.77 (15.38–50.00)	25.00 (11.76–46.15)	38.46 (20.00–53.85)	
Mean ± SD	34.13 ± 23.65	31.25 ± 22.44	40.81 ± 25.06	
Max core involvement, %				
Median (IQR)	70.0 (30.0–85.0)	60.0 (30.0–85.0)	85.0 (50.0–85.0)	
Mean ± SD	58.68 ± 30.19	55.66 ± 30.48	65.71 ± 28.37	
Clinical T stage, n (%)				<0.001 *
T1	58 (10.8)	28 (7.5)	30 (18.6)	
T2	477 (89.2)	346 (92.5)	131 (81.4)	
Pathological T stage, n (%)				<0.001 *
T2	273 (51.0)	215 (57.5)	58 (36.0)	
T3	262 (49.0)	159 (42.5)	103 (64.0)	
Postoperative pathology, n (%)				
Positive surgical margin	161 (30.1)	61 (16.3)	100 (62.1)	<0.001 *
Extracapsular extension	274 (51.2)	159 (42.5)	115 (71.4)	<0.001 *
Seminal vesicle invasion	90 (17.0)	57 (15.2)	33 (20.5)	0.136
Lymph nodal metastasis	10 (1.9)	7 (1.9)	3 (1.9)	0.346

NAPCa—non-apex prostate cancer; APCa—apex prostate cancer; IQR—interquartile range; SD—standard deviation; BMI—body mass index; PSA—prostate-specific antigen; DRE—digital rectal examination; GG—grading group; RP—radical prostatectomy; PSAD; prostate-specific antigen density. * statistically significant.

Table 2. Univariate and multivariate analysis for predicting GG upgrading.

	Univariate		Multivariate	
	OR (95% CI)	*p* Value	OR (95% CI)	*p* Value
(a) All patients (n = 535)				
Age, years	1.018 (0.992–1.045)	0.165	1.022 (0.996–1.050)	0.103
BMI, kg/m^2	0.971 (0.915–1.031)	0.333	0.992 (0.933–1.055)	0.794
Serum PSA, ng/mL	1.018 (1.003–1.033)	0.018 *	-	-
Prostate volume, mL	0.987 (0.989–1.000)	0.066	-	-
PSAD, ng/mL^2	3.164 (1.743–5.744)	<0.001 *	4.149 (2.151–8.001)	<0.001 *
Number of biopsy cores	0.978 (0.925–1.034)	0.432	-	
Percent positive biopsy cores, %	0.734 (0.356–1.513)	0.403	0.488 (0.185–1.285)	0.146
Max core involvement, %	0.997 (0.991–1.003)	0.307	0.997 (0.989–1.004)	0.346
(b) Non-apex prostate cancer (n = 374)				
Age, years	1.015 (0.982–1.048)	0.383	1.016 (0.982–1.051)	0.365
BMI, kg/m^2	0.968 (0.902–1.040)	0.377	0.999 (0.928–1.077)	0.988
Serum PSA, ng/mL	1.021 (1.000–1.043)	0.046 *	-	-
Prostate volume, mL	0.991 (0.983–0.999)	0.035 *	-	-
PSAD, ng/mL^2	5.429 (2.378–12.397)	<0.001 *	8.176 (3.288–20.331)	<0.001 *
Number of biopsy cores	0.970 (0.904–1.041)	0.401	-	
Percent positive biopsy cores, %	0.639 (0.255–1.597)	0.338	0.371 (0.105–1.305)	0.122
Max core involvement, %	0.996 (0.989–1.003)	0.229	0.995 (0.986–1.003)	0.228
(c) Apex prostate cancer (n = 161)				
Age, years	1.026 (0.982–1.071)	0.250	1.031 (0.987–1.078)	0.171
BMI, kg/m^2	0.969 (0.866–1.084)	0.578	0.970 (0.866–1.088)	0.606
Serum PSA, ng/mL	1.014 (0.992–1.036)	0.230	-	-
Prostate volume, mL	1.000 (0.986–1.014)	0.970	-	-
PSAD, ng/mL^2	1.332 (0.516–3.436)	0.554	1.468 (0.528–4.079)	0.462
Number of biopsy cores	0.981 (0.892–1.079)	0.697	-	
Percent positive biopsy cores, %	0.811 (0.235–2.802)	0.741	0.699 (0.143–3.421)	0.658
Max core involvement, %	0.999 (0.988–1.010)	0.843	0.999 (0.986–1.013)	0.910

OR—odds ratio; BMI—body mass index; PSAD—prostate-specific antigen. * statistically significant.

There were 262 patients (49.0%) who had pathological upstaging after RP. However, no significant differences in age ($p = 0.359$), BMI ($p = 0.110$), or number of biopsy cores ($p = 0.809$) were observed (Table S1). The univariate analysis showed that higher PSA (OR: 1.035, $p < 0.001$), smaller PV (OR: 0.980, $p < 0.001$), higher PSAD (OR: 7.244, $p < 0.001$), higher number of positive cores (OR: 1.232, $p < 0.001$), higher percentage of positive cores (OR: 15.821, $p < 0.001$), and higher max core involvement (OR: 1.018, $p < 0.001$) were predictive of pathological upstaging. The multivariable analysis revealed that both PSAD (OR: 4.750, $p < 0.001$) and percentage of positive cores (OR: 5.108, $p = 0.002$) were independent, significant predictors of upstaging (Table 3).

3.3. The Patients with NAPCa

Of the 374 patients with NAPCa, 168 (44.9%) had GG upgrading after RP. Serum PSA ($p = 0.001$) and PSAD ($p < 0.001$) were significantly higher in upgraded patients than in non-upgraded patients. There were no significant differences in age ($p = 0.506$), BMI ($p = 0.423$), PV ($p = 0.068$), number of biopsy cores ($p = 0.416$), number of positive cores ($p = 0.414$), percentage of positive cores ($p = 0.610$), and max core involvement ($p = 0.324$) (Table S2). The univariate analysis showed that serum PSA (OR: 1.021, $p = 0.046$), PV (OR: 0.991, $p = 0.035$), and PSAD (OR: 5.429, $p < 0.001$) were significant predictors of GG upgrading. The multivariate analysis showed that PSAD (OR: 8.176, $p < 0.001$) was an independent predictor of GG upgrading (Table 2).

Table 3. Univariate and multivariate analysis for predicting pathological upstaging.

	Univariate		Multivariate	
	OR (95% CI)	***p* Value**	**OR (95% CI)**	***p* Value**
(a) All patients (n = 535)				
Age, years	1.013 (0.987–1.039)	0.334	1.014 (0.986–1.043)	0.329
BMI, kg/m^2	1.049 (0.988–1.113)	0.118	1.063 (0.996–1.134)	0.064
Serum PSA, ng/ml	1.035 (1.017–1.053)	<0.001 *	-	-
Prostate volume, ml	0.980 (0.972–0.988)	<0.001 *	-	-
PSAD, ng/mL^2	7.244 (3.556–14.755)	<0.001 *	4.750 (2.259–9.984)	<0.001 *
Number of biopsy cores	1.232 (1.158–1.311)	<0.001 *	-	
Percent positive biopsy cores, %	15.821 (7.011–35.700)	<0.001 *	5.108 (1.854–14.074)	0.002 *
Max core involvement, %	1.018 (1.012–1.024)	<0.001 *	1.007 (1.000–1.015)	0.051
(b) Non-apex prostate cancer (n = 374)				
Age, years	1.009 (0.977–1.043)	0.568	1.009 (0.972–1.046)	0.645
BMI, kg/m^2	1.040 (0.968–1.117)	0.287	1.056 (0.977–1.142)	0.171
Serum PSA, ng/mL	1.034 (1.009–1.059)	0.007 *	-	-
Prostate volume, mL	0.973 (0.962–0.984)	<0.001 *	-	-
PSAD, ng/mL^2	7.142 (3.031–16.830)	<0.001 *	4.973 (1.996–12.391)	0.001 *
Number of biopsy cores	1.238 (1.146–1.336)	<0.001 *	-	
Percent positive biopsy cores, %	15.651 (5.733–42.727)	<0.001 *	3.994 (1.108–14.399)	0.034 *
Max core involvement, %	1.017 (1.009–1.024)	<0.001 *	1.006 (0.997–1.015)	0.199
(c) Apex prostate cancer (n = 161)				
Age, years	1.021 (0.977–1.067)	0.352	1.022 (0.976–1.070)	0.361
BMI, kg/m^2	1.015 (0.904–1.141)	0.800	1.038 (0.918–1.175)	0.551
Serum PSA, ng/mL	1.044 (1.005–1.085)	0.027 *	-	-
Prostate volume, mL	0.989 (0.975–1.004)	0.142	-	-
PSAD, ng/mL/cm^3	4.063 (1.169–14.120)	0.027 *	2.906 (0.816–10.342)	0.100
Number of biopsy cores	1.171 (1.048–1.307)	0.005 *	-	
Percent positive biopsy cores, %	8.920 (2.105–37.807)	0.003 *	3.489 (0.576–21.142)	0.174
Max core involvement, %	1.016 (1.004–1.028)	0.007 *	1.009 (0.994–1.023)	0.236

OR—odds ratio; BMI—body mass index; PSAD—prostate-specific antigen. * statistically significant.

Pathological upstaging occurred in 159 (42.5%) patients with NAPCa. Upstaged patients had higher PSA ($p < 0.001$), smaller PV ($p < 0.001$), higher PSAD ($p < 0.001$), a higher percentage of positive cores ($p < 0.001$), and higher max core involvement ($p = 0.007$). No statistically significant differences were found in age ($p = 0.694$), BMI ($p = 0.293$), or number of biopsy cores ($p = 0.574$) (Table S2). Univariate analysis revealed that higher PSA (OR: 1.034, $p = 0.007$), lower PV (OR: 0.973, $p < 0.001$), higher PSAD (OR: 7.142, $p < 0.001$), higher number of positive cores (OR: 1.238, $p < 0.001$), higher percentage of positive cores (OR: 15.651, $p < 0.001$), and higher max core involvement (OR: 1.017, $p < 0.001$) were predictive of upstaging. In the multivariate analysis, PSAD (OR: 4.973, $p = 0.001$) and percentage of positive cores (OR: 3.994, $p = 0.034$) were independently predictive of pathological upstaging (Table 3).

3.4. The Patients with APCa

Of the 161 patients with APCa, 77 (47.8%) were identified as having GG upgrading after RP. Serum PSA ($p = 0.024$) was significantly higher in patients with GG upgrading than those who did not present GG upgrading. No statistically significant differences were found in age ($p = 0.215$), BMI ($p = 0.647$), PV ($p = 0.929$), PSAD ($p = 0.182$), number of biopsy cores ($p = 0.633$), percentage of positive cores ($p = 0.764$) and max core involvement ($p = 0.642$) (Table S3). The univariate and multivariate analysis revealed that age ($p = 0.171$), BMI ($p = 0.606$), PSAD ($p = 0.462$), percentage of positive cores ($p = 0.658$), and max core involvement ($p = 0.910$) were not independently associated with GG upgrading (Table 2).

There were 103 (64.0%) patients with pathological upstaging. Upstaged patients had higher PSA ($p < 0.001$), higher PSAD ($p = 0.002$), higher percentage positive cores

(p = 0.005), and higher max core involvement (p = 0.005) compared with those who did not display upstaging. There were no statistically significant differences in age (p = 0.384), BMI (p = 0.665), PV (p = 0.146) or number of biopsy cores (p = 0.237) (Table S3). Univariate analysis revealed that higher PSA (OR: 1.044, p = 0.027), higher PSAD (OR: 4.063, p = 0.027), higher number of positive cores (OR: 1.171, p = 0.005), higher percentage of positive cores (OR: 8.920, p = 0.003), and higher max core involvement (OR: 1.016, p = 0.007) were predictors of upstaging. However, there were no independent, significant predictors, including PSAD (p = 0.100), for predicting pathological upstaging in multivariate analysis (Table 3).

3.5. Predictive Characteristics of PSAD

Of the entire cohort, the AUC value of PSAD for predicting GG upgrading was 0.637 (95% CI: 0.595–0.678, p < 0.001). The cut-off value of 0.23 ng/mL^2 showed a sensitivity of 68.98%, specificity of 53.45%, a positive predictive value (PPV) of 55.59%, and a negative predictive value (NPV) of 67.10%. The AUC value of PSAD for predicting upstaging in all patients was 0.737 (95% CI: 0.698–0.774, p < 0.001). A cut-off value of 0.23 ng/mL^2 showed a sensitivity of 77.86%, specificity of 62.27%, a PPV of 66.45%, and a NPV of 74.56% (Table 4).

Table 4. The predictive characteristics of PSAD for predicting upgrading and upstaging.

	AUC (95% CI)	Cutoff, ng/mL^2	Sensitivity (%)	Specificity (%)	PPV (%)	NPV (%)
(a) All patients (n = 535)						
Upgrading	0.637 (0.595–0.678)	0.23	68.98	53.45	55.59	67.10
Upstaging	0.737 (0.698–0.774)	0.23	77.86	62.27	66.45	74.56
(b) Non-apex prostate cancer (n = 374)						
Upgrading	0.670 (0.620−0.718)	0.17	85.71	41.75	54.53	78.19
Upstaging	0.775 (0.729−0.816)	0.23	79.25	66.98	63.95	81.37

PSAD—prostate-specific antigen; AUC—area under the curve; CI—confidence interval; PPV—positive predictive value; NPV—negative predictive value.

Of the 374 patients with NAPCa, the AUC value of PSAD for predicting GG upgrading was 0.670 (95% CI: 0.620–0.718, p < 0.001). A cut-off value of 0.17 ng/mL^2 showed a sensitivity of 85.71%, a specificity of 41.75%, a PPV of 54.53%, and a NPV of 78.19%. The AUC value of PSAD for predicting upstaging in patients with NAPCa was 0.775 (95% CI: 0.729–0.816, p < 0.001). A cut-off value of 0.23 ng/mL^2 showed a sensitivity of 79.25%, specificity of 66.98%, a PPV of 63.95%, and a NPV of 81.37% (Table 4).

4. Discussion

It is well established that biopsy GG and clinical T stage contribute the most to estimating the prognosis of PCa [15]. However, pathological GG upgrading and upstaging from biopsy to RP specimens is quite common. According to prior studies, the rate of GG upgrading at RP varies from 30% to 50%, meaning that nearly half of all biopsy sampling does not reflect the overall pathological characteristics of prostate specimens [5,16,17]. Furthermore, Gleason GG upgrading and pathological upstaging have been associated with adverse outcomes, including unfavorable pathological features and biochemical recurrence [10]. In the current study, GG upgrading and pathological upstaging after RP were recorded in 45.8% and 49.0% of patients, respectively. Although the definition of upgrading and upstaging may be different between studies, the current results showed a relatively higher rate than those of other reports. This may be because more than one-third of the patients (34.2%, 183/535) in our study were in intermediate or high-risk groups according to D'Amico classification, and the median PSA value was 10.93 ng/mL. Thus, the patients' characteristics in this cohort were relatively more aggressive than those in other studies. Furthermore, the lack of multi-parametric magnetic resonance imaging (mpMRI) findings, especially in multifocal tumors, may explain the relatively high proportion of patients with GG upgrading at post-RP, as well as the poor performance of biopsy.

Systematic TRUS-guided prostate biopsy has been widely accepted as a mainstay in the diagnosis of PCa, whether it occurs via the transrectal or transperineal approach [15]. Despite the use of appropriate techniques, this method has been shown to underestimate the presence of malignant disease, with false-negative rates ranging from 20% to 40% [18]. The reasons for this occurrence may differ based on tumor location. Particularly in the apex, the occupied volume is very small, and the angle attained by the transrectal approach might be quite limited. It should be noted that the transrectal approach more easily misses tumors located at the apex region. In the current study, all patients underwent TRUS-guided prostate biopsy through the transrectal route. After analysis of the RP specimens, APCa was found in 30.1% (161/535) of patients. In addition, patients with APCa were associated with adverse pathological characteristics. Ishii et al. reported a 36% rate of PCa located predominantly in the apex, and the frequency increased over time [19]. The current results confirmed this previous finding. However, Sazuka et al. demonstrated that in Japanese patients, the apex was the area of cancer most frequently identified (85%), and the section false-negative rate was 45% for transrectal biopsy [20]. These findings suggested that there may be geographic and racial differences in PCa localization.

It is well known that PSAD was initially introduced to improve the accuracy of the PSA test for PCa screening. Several studies have observed that PSAD is significantly better than PSA alone at predicting adverse pathology and biochemical recurrence after RP [12]. The current results also indicate that PSAD may be an effective predictor of adverse pathological features in the entire study cohort (data not shown). Nonetheless, Jones et al. were unable to demonstrate that PSAD outperformed PSA in assessing early biochemical recurrence [21]. Other studies have reported that PSA is more accurate than PSAD in predicting total tumor volume and biochemical recurrence [22]. The discrepancy between those results and the current study may be due to various factors, including differences in tumor location and biopsy schemes between different studies.

Recently, the National Comprehensive Cancer Network guideline has adopted PSAD as an inclusion criterion for active surveillance (AS) in patients with PCa [23]. Ha et al. also demonstrated that removing PSAD from the AS criterion would significantly increase the rate of pathological upgrading and upstaging [24]. However, the association between PSAD and pathological GG upgrading in patients with PCa still remains elusive. In one study, Brassetti et al. recently proved that PSAD is a valuable predictor of upgrading and upstaging in candidates for surgery or AS [25]. Furthermore, Sim et al. also reported that magnetic resonance imaging-based PSAD > 0.26 ng/mL^2 could aid in the prediction of postoperative upgrading in patients with low-risk PCa [26]. In addition, the specificity and PPV were both relatively high (84.9% and 83.3%, respectively). Nonetheless, Keefe et al. demonstrated that in PCa with a biopsy-proven GS 3 + 4 = 7, clinicopathological features including PSAD were not significantly related to upgrading or upstaging [27]. Ning et al. did not find a significant correlation between PSAD and upgrading using multivariate analysis [28].

Recently, mpMRI of the prostate has increasingly utilized to diagnosis, staging, and risk stratification of PCa [29]. Several systematic reviews have reported that pooled NPVs in the detection of clinically significant PCa for mpMRI ranged from 88% to 93%, with a consequent optimization of the reduction of unnecessary biopsy or overtreatment [30,31]. It is well documented that including mpMRI in an AS cohort may improve the ability to predict GG upgrading. Mamawala et al. showed that mpMRI was an independent predictive factor for GG upgrading in follow-up AS biopsy [32]. However, Chu et al. demonstrated that mpMRI alone was insufficient to detect GG upgrading on AS, especially among patients with PSAD $\geq$ 0.15 ng/mL^2 [33]. Meanwhile, Christiansen et al. reported that PSAD was of clinical importance for predicting GG upgrading in patients with PI-RADS 4–5, whereas for men with PI-RADS 4–5, the probability of upgrading was high, regardless of PSAD [34].

Thus, incorporating mpMRI and other clinicopathological parameters including PSAD may overcome the limitations and improve diagnostic accuracy for prediction upgrading.

In the present study, PSAD was an independent, significant predictor of GG upgrading and pathological upstaging when all patients in the cohort were analyzed. The cut-off value proposed for the prediction of GG upgrading was 0.23 ng/mL^2, but the performance accuracy of PSAD was unsatisfactory, with an AUC value of 63.7%. The sensitivity, specificity, PPV, and NPV were 68.98%, 53.45%, 55.59%, and 67.10%, respectively, which is inferior compared to other studies. Potential confounders include the disadvantages of the biopsy scheme and tumor location in the prostate, which were likely related to limited efficiency in predicting upgrading. Interestingly, after classifying the cohort into APCa and NAPCa groups based on whether the tumor existed in the apex, PSAD only remained significantly associated with Gleason GG upgrading and pathological upstaging in NAPCa patients and was not significant in patients with APCa. In addition, the AUC value of PSAD for predicting GG upgrading in NAPCa patients was 67.0%, with no significant difference before and after classification. However, the sensitivity, specificity, PPV and NPV increased remarkably after grouping, with values of 85.71%, 41.75%, 54.53%, and 78.19%, respectively.

These results suggest that more attention should be paid to the tumor location, especially with regard to the apex region, which might lead to inaccurate biopsy GG evaluation and incorrect analysis. Men with APCa might not benefit from the use of PSAD to predict GG upgrading and pathological upstaging after RP. One possible reason is that all patients in the cohort did not receive an apex-targeted biopsy in the systematic prostate biopsy, and thus small, aggressive PCa with a higher GG at the apex region might be missed. Several studies have demonstrated that adding apex cores improved the detection rate of clinically significant PCa (GS $\geq$ 7), particularly in early stage disease [35,36]. Therefore, it is especially important in patients with low-risk PCa who seek less invasive therapy, such as watchful waiting and AS, to additionally target the apex region during systematic biopsy. This may help to precisely select patients for AS protocols. Furthermore, comprehensive consideration of PSAD and cancer location may be more reasonable for patient counseling and clinical decision making. Additional sampling of biopsy cores from the apex region may help improve the accuracy of PSAD in predicting GG upgrading and pathological upstaging after RP.

There are several limitations of this study, including its retrospective design and relatively small number of patients. First, there was no systematic, pathological review of all specimens, although the interobserver variability is well known. Second, all patients analyzed in this study underwent TRUS-guided core biopsies without multi-parameter MRI. Multi-parameter MRI focusing on the prostatic apex was superior to systematic biopsy for identifying adverse APCa [37]. In addition, several studies have demonstrated that MRI targeted fusion biopsy could enhance the diagnostic accuracy of PCa detection in final histopathology, with a lower rate of upgrading than TRUS-guided biopsy [3,28]. In this regard, the rate of PCa detection in the current study could have been underestimated, while the rate of upgraded GG could have been overestimated. Third, our study also has a lack of genomic classifiers such as the Oncotype DX Genomic Prostate Score test, which has been reported to be associated with biopsy upgrading [38,39]. Furthermore, the study focus was primarily on the pathological findings. Biochemical recurrence and PCa-specific mortality were not evaluated; these may be more crucial issues than adverse pathological features for better defining tumor progression.

5. Conclusions

PSAD may aid in the prediction of GG upgrading and pathological upstaging in patients with PCa. However, this advantage may only be practical in patients with NAPCa identified after RP. Additional biopsy cores taken from the prostatic apex region may help improve the accuracy of PSAD in predicting pathological GG upgrading and upstaging after RP.

Supplementary Materials: The following supporting information can be downloaded at: https://www.mdpi.com/article/10.3390/jcm12041659/s1, Table S1: Comparison of upgrading and upstaging in all of patients (n = 535); Table S2: Comparison of upgrading and upstaging in patients with NAPCa (n = 374); Table S3: Comparison of upgrading and upstaging in patients with APCa (n = 161).

Author Contributions: Conceptualization, C.H. and G.S.; methodology, C.H.; software, S.H.; validation, Q.H. and L.Z.; formal analysis, L.Z.; investigation, C.H.; resources, L.Z.; data curation, Y.G.; writing—original draft preparation, C.H.; writing—review and editing, G.S.; visualization, C.H.; supervision, G.S. and L.Z.; project administration, G.S. and L.Z.; funding acquisition, L.Z. All authors have read and agreed to the published version of the manuscript.

Funding: This research was funded by National Natural Science Foundation of China (grant number: 81972379, 82173216, 81872083, and 81972380), the Capital Health Research and Development of Special (grant number: 2022-1-4072), the Clinical Features Research of Capital (grant number: Z211100002921070), Clinical Medicine Plus X—Young Scholars Project, Peking University, the Fundamental Research Funds for the Central Universities (grant number: PKU2021LCXQ026) and Wuxi "Taihu Talents Program" Medical and Health High-level Talents Project.

Institutional Review Board Statement: The study was conducted in accordance with the Declaration of Helsinki, and approved by the Ethics Committee of Peking University First Hospital (protocol code 2018-177 and date of approval 31 August 2018).

Informed Consent Statement: Patient consent was waived due to the retrospective nature of the study.

Data Availability Statement: Not applicable.

Conflicts of Interest: The authors declare no conflict of interest.

References

1. Siegel, R.L.; Miller, K.D.; Jemal, A. Cancer statistics, 2018. *CA Cancer J. Clin.* **2018**, *68*, 7–30. [CrossRef] [PubMed]
2. Athanazio, D.; Gotto, G.; Shea-Budgell, M.; Yilmaz, A.; Trpkov, K. Global Gleason grade groups in prostate cancer: Concordance of biopsy and radical prostatectomy grades and predictors of upgrade and downgrade. *Histopathology* **2017**, *70*, 1098–1106. [CrossRef] [PubMed]
3. Calio, B.P.; Sidana, A.; Sugano, D.; Gaur, S.; Maruf, M.; Jain, A.L.; Merino, M.J.; Choyke, P.L.; Wood, B.J.; Pinto, P.A.; et al. Risk of Upgrading from Prostate Biopsy to Radical Prostatectomy Pathology-Does Saturation Biopsy of Index Lesion during Multiparametric Magnetic Resonance Imaging-Transrectal Ultrasound Fusion Biopsy Help? *J. Urol.* **2018**, *199*, 976–982. [CrossRef] [PubMed]
4. D'Amico, A.V.; Whittington, R.; Malkowicz, S.B.; Schultz, D.; Blank, K.; Broderick, G.A.; Tomaszewski, J.E.; Renshaw, A.A.; Kaplan, I.; Beard, C.J.; et al. Biochemical outcome after radical prostatectomy, external beam radiation therapy, or interstitial radiation therapy for clinically localized prostate cancer. *JAMA* **1998**, *280*, 969–974. [CrossRef]
5. Epstein, J.I.; Feng, Z.; Trock, B.J.; Pierorazio, P.M. Upgrading and downgrading of prostate cancer from biopsy to radical prostatectomy: Incidence and predictive factors using the modified Gleason grading system and factoring in tertiary grades. *Eur. Urol.* **2012**, *61*, 1019–1024. [CrossRef]
6. Epstein, J.I.; Egevad, L.; Amin, M.B.; Delahunt, B.; Srigley, J.R.; Humphrey, P.A.; Grading, C. The 2014 International Society of Urological Pathology (ISUP) Consensus Conference on Gleason Grading of Prostatic Carcinoma: Definition of Grading Patterns and Proposal for a New Grading System. *Am. J. Surg. Pathol.* **2016**, *40*, 244–252. [CrossRef]
7. Humphrey, P.A.; Moch, H.; Cubilla, A.L.; Ulbright, T.M.; Reuter, V.E. The 2016 WHO Classification of Tumours of the Urinary System and Male Genital Organs-Part B: Prostate and Bladder Tumours. *Eur. Urol.* **2016**, *70*, 106–119. [CrossRef]
8. Loeb, S.; Folkvaljon, Y.; Robinson, D.; Lissbrant, I.F.; Egevad, L.; Stattin, P. Evaluation of the 2015 Gleason Grade Groups in a Nationwide Population-based Cohort. *Eur. Urol.* **2016**, *69*, 1135–1141. [CrossRef]
9. Iremashvili, V.; Pelaez, L.; Jorda, M.; Manoharan, M.; Arianayagam, M.; Rosenberg, D.L.; Soloway, M.S. Prostate sampling by 12-core biopsy: Comparison of the biopsy results with tumor location in prostatectomy specimens. *Urology* **2012**, *79*, 37–42. [CrossRef]
10. Magheli, A.; Rais-Bahrami, S.; Trock, B.J.; Humphreys, E.B.; Partin, A.W.; Han, M.; Gonzalgo, M.L. Prostate specific antigen versus prostate specific antigen density as a prognosticator of pathological characteristics and biochemical recurrence following radical prostatectomy. *J. Urol.* **2008**, *179*, 1780–1784. [CrossRef]
11. Mitsuzuka, K.; Narita, S.; Koie, T.; Kaiho, Y.; Tsuchiya, N.; Yoneyama, T.; Kakoi, N.; Kawamura, S.; Tochigi, T.; Habuchi, T.; et al. Pathological and biochemical outcomes after radical prostatectomy in men with low-risk prostate cancer meeting the Prostate Cancer International: Active Surveillance criteria. *BJU Int.* **2013**, *111*, 914–920. [CrossRef]

12. Oh, J.J.; Hong, S.K.; Lee, J.K.; Lee, B.K.; Lee, S.; Kwon, O.S.; Byun, S.S.; Lee, S.E. Prostate-specific antigen vs prostate-specific antigen density as a predictor of upgrading in men diagnosed with Gleason 6 prostate cancer by contemporary multicore prostate biopsy. *BJU Int.* **2012**, *110*, E494–E499. [CrossRef] [PubMed]
13. de Cobelli, O.; Terracciano, D.; Tagliabue, E.; Raimondi, S.; Galasso, G.; Cioffi, A.; Cordima, G.; Musi, G.; Damiano, R.; Cantiello, F.; et al. Body mass index was associated with upstaging and upgrading in patients with low-risk prostate cancer who met the inclusion criteria for active surveillance. *Urol. Oncol.* **2015**, *33*, 201.e1–201.e8. [CrossRef] [PubMed]
14. Samaratunga, H.; Montironi, R.; True, L.; Epstein, J.I.; Griffiths, D.F.; Humphrey, P.A.; van der Kwast, T.; Wheeler, T.M.; Srigley, J.R.; Delahunt, B.; et al. International Society of Urological Pathology (ISUP) Consensus Conference on Handling and Staging of Radical Prostatectomy Specimens. Working group 1: Specimen handling. *Mod. Pathol.* **2011**, *24*, 6–15. [CrossRef] [PubMed]
15. Mottet, N.; Bellmunt, J.; Bolla, M.; Briers, E.; Cumberbatch, M.G.; De Santis, M.; Fossati, N.; Gross, T.; Henry, A.M.; Joniau, S.; et al. EAU-ESTRO-SIOG Guidelines on Prostate Cancer. Part 1: Screening, Diagnosis, and Local Treatment with Curative Intent. *Eur. Urol.* **2017**, *71*, 618–629. [CrossRef]
16. Thomas, C.; Pfirrmann, K.; Pieles, F.; Bogumil, A.; Gillitzer, R.; Wiesner, C.; Thuroff, J.W.; Melchior, S.W. Predictors for clinically relevant Gleason score upgrade in patients undergoing radical prostatectomy. *BJU Int.* **2012**, *109*, 214–219. [CrossRef]
17. Cosimo, N.; Aldo, B.; Giuseppe, S.; Riccardo, L.; Riccardo, M.; Devis, C.; Giovanni, M.; Michele, G.; Andrea, T. Metabolic syndrome increases the risk of upgrading and upstaging in patients with prostate cancer on biopsy: A radical prostatectomy multicenter cohort study. *Prostate Cancer Prostatic Dis.* **2018**, *21*, 438–445. [CrossRef]
18. Bjurlin, M.A.; Taneja, S.S. Standards for prostate biopsy. *Curr. Opin. Urol.* **2014**, *24*, 155–161. [CrossRef]
19. Ishii, J.; Ohori, M.; Scardino, P.; Tsuboi, T.; Slawin, K.; Wheeler, T. Significance of the craniocaudal distribution of cancer in radical prostatectomy specimens. *Int. J. Urol.* **2007**, *14*, 817–821. [CrossRef]
20. Sazuka, T.; Imamoto, T.; Namekawa, T.; Utsumi, T.; Yanagisawa, M.; Kawamura, K.; Kamiya, N.; Suzuki, H.; Ueda, T.; Ota, S.; et al. Analysis of preoperative detection for apex prostate cancer by transrectal biopsy. *Prostate Cancer* **2013**, *2013*, 705865. [CrossRef]
21. Jones, T.D.; Koch, M.O.; Bunde, P.J.; Cheng, L. Is prostate-specific antigen (PSA) density better than the preoperative PSA level in predicting early biochemical recurrence of prostate cancer after radical prostatectomy? *BJU Int.* **2006**, *97*, 480–484. [CrossRef]
22. Brassell, S.A.; Kao, T.C.; Sun, L.; Moul, J.W. Prostate-specific antigen versus prostate-specific antigen density as predictor of tumor volume, margin status, pathologic stage, and biochemical recurrence of prostate cancer. *Urology* **2005**, *66*, 1229–1233. [CrossRef] [PubMed]
23. Mohler, J.; Bahnson, R.R.; Boston, B.; Busby, J.E.; D'Amico, A.; Eastham, J.A.; Enke, C.A.; George, D.; Horwitz, E.M.; Huben, R.P.; et al. NCCN clinical practice guidelines in oncology: Prostate cancer. *J. Natl. Compr. Canc. Netw.* **2010**, *8*, 162–200. [CrossRef] [PubMed]
24. Ha, Y.S.; Yu, J.; Salmasi, A.H.; Patel, N.; Parihar, J.; Singer, E.A.; Kim, J.H.; Kwon, T.G.; Kim, W.J.; Kim, I.Y. Prostate-specific antigen density toward a better cutoff to identify better candidates for active surveillance. *Urology* **2014**, *84*, 365–371. [CrossRef]
25. Brassetti, A.; Lombardo, R.; Emiliozzi, P.; Cardi, A.; Antonio, V.; Antonio, I.; Aldo, S.; Tommaso, R.; Alberto, P.; Gianluca, D. Prostate-specific Antigen Density Is a Good Predictor of Upstaging and Upgrading, According to the New Grading System: The Keys We Are Seeking May Be Already in Our Pocket. *Urology* **2018**, *111*, 129–135. [CrossRef]
26. Sim, K.C.; Sung, D.J.; Kang, K.W.; Yang, K.S.; Han, N.Y.; Park, B.J.; Kim, M.J.; Cho, S.B. Magnetic Resonance Imaging-Based Prostate-Specific Antigen Density for Prediction of Gleason Score Upgrade in Patients With Low-Risk Prostate Cancer on Initial Biopsy. *J. Comput. Assist. Tomogr.* **2017**, *41*, 731–736. [CrossRef] [PubMed]
27. Keefe, D.T.; Schieda, N.; El Hallani, S.; Breau, R.H.; Morash, C.; Robertson, S.J.; Mai, K.T.; Belanger, E.C.; Flood, T.A. Cribriform morphology predicts upstaging after radical prostatectomy in patients with Gleason score 3 + 4 = 7 prostate cancer at transrectal ultrasound (TRUS)-guided needle biopsy. *Virchows Arch.* **2015**, *467*, 437–442. [CrossRef]
28. Xu, N.; Wu, Y.P.; Li, X.D.; Lin, M.Y.; Zheng, Q.S.; Chen, S.H.; Li, J.F.; Wei, Y.; Xue, X.Y. Risk of upgrading from prostate biopsy to radical prostatectomy pathology: Is magnetic resonance imaging-guided biopsy more accurate? *J. Cancer* **2018**, *9*, 3634–3639. [CrossRef]
29. Stabile, A.; Giganti, F.; Rosenkrantz, A.B.; Taneja, S.S.; Villeirs, G.; Gill, I.S.; Allen, C.; Emberton, M.; Moore, C.M.; Kasivisvanathan, V. Multiparametric MRI for prostate cancer diagnosis: Current status and future directions. *Nat. Rev. Urol.* **2020**, *17*, 41–61. [CrossRef]
30. Sathianathen, N.J.; Omer, A.; Harriss, E.; Davies, L.; Kasivisvanathan, V.; Punwani, S.; Moore, C.M.; Kastner, C.; Barrett, T.; Van Den Bergh, R.C.; et al. Negative Predictive Value of Multiparametric Magnetic Resonance Imaging in the Detection of Clinically Significant Prostate Cancer in the Prostate Imaging Reporting and Data System Era: A Systematic Review and Meta-analysis. *Eur. Urol.* **2020**, *78*, 402–414. [CrossRef]
31. Moldovan, P.C.; Van den Broeck, T.; Sylvester, R.; Marconi, L.; Bellmunt, J.; van den Bergh, R.C.N.; Bolla, M.; Briers, E.; Cumberbatch, M.G.; Fossati, N.; et al. What Is the Negative Predictive Value of Multiparametric Magnetic Resonance Imaging in Excluding Prostate Cancer at Biopsy? A Systematic Review and Meta-analysis from the European Association of Urology Prostate Cancer Guidelines Panel. *Eur. Urol.* **2017**, *72*, 250–266. [CrossRef]
32. Mamawala, M.K.; Meyer, A.R.; Landis, P.K.; Macura, K.J.; Epstein, J.I.; Partin, A.W.; Carter, B.H.; Gorin, M.A. Utility of multiparametric magnetic resonance imaging in the risk stratification of men with Grade Group 1 prostate cancer on active surveillance. *BJU Int.* **2020**, *125*, 861–866. [CrossRef] [PubMed]

33. Chu, C.E.; Lonergan, P.E.; Washington, S.L.; Cowan, J.E.; Shinohara, K.; Westphalen, A.C.; Carroll, P.R.; Cooperberg, M.R. Multiparametric Magnetic Resonance Imaging Alone is Insufficient to Detect Grade Reclassification in Active Surveillance for Prostate Cancer. *Eur. Urol.* **2020**, *78*, 515–517. [CrossRef] [PubMed]
34. Christiansen, O.; Bratt, O.; Kirkevold, O.; Benth, J.S.; Manoharan, P.; Selnes, A.; Haug, E.S.; Slaaen, M. Predictors of upgrading from low-grade cancer at prostatectomy in men with biparametric magnetic resonance imaging. *Cent. Eur. J. Urol.* **2022**, *75*, 35–40. [CrossRef]
35. Moussa, A.S.; Meshref, A.; Schoenfield, L.; Masoud, A.; Abdel-Rahman, S.; Li, J.; Flazoura, S.; Magi-Galluzzi, C.; Fergany, A.; Fareed, K.; et al. Importance of additional "extreme" anterior apical needle biopsies in the initial detection of prostate cancer. *Urology* **2010**, *75*, 1034–1039. [CrossRef] [PubMed]
36. Elshafei, A.; Kartha, G.; Li, Y.; Moussa, A.S.; Hatem, A.; Gao, T.; Jones, J.S. Low risk patients benefit from extreme anterior apical sampling on initial biopsy for prostate cancer diagnosis. *Prostate* **2014**, *74*, 1183–1188. [CrossRef]
37. Kenigsberg, A.P.; Tamada, T.; Rosenkrantz, A.B.; Llukani, E.; Deng, F.M.; Melamed, J.; Zhou, M.; Lepor, H. Multiparametric magnetic resonance imaging identifies significant apical prostate cancers. *BJU Int.* **2018**, *121*, 239–243. [CrossRef]
38. Cedars, B.E.; Washington, S.L.; Cowan, J.E.; Leapman, M.; Tenggara, I.; Chan, J.M.; Cooperberg, M.R.; Carroll, P.R. Stability of a 17-Gene Genomic Prostate Score in Serial Testing of Men on Active Surveillance for Early Stage Prostate Cancer. *J. Urol.* **2019**, *202*, 696–701. [CrossRef]
39. Kornberg, Z.; Cowan, J.E.; Westphalen, A.C.; Cooperberg, M.R.; Chan, J.M.; Zhao, S.; Shinohara, K.; Carroll, P.R. Genomic Prostate Score, PI-RADS version 2 and Progression in Men with Prostate Cancer on Active Surveillance. *J. Urol.* **2019**, *201*, 300–307. [CrossRef]

MDPI AG
Grosspeteranlage 5
4052 Basel
Switzerland
Tel.: +41 61 683 77 34

Journal of Clinical Medicine Editorial Office
E-mail: jcm@mdpi.com
www.mdpi.com/journal/jcm

www.ingramcontent.com/pod-product-compliance
Lightning Source LLC
Chambersburg PA
CBHW041340210926
51850CB00013B/2937
* 9 7 8 3 7 2 5 8 4 2 9 5 7 *